Tasty

A CURIOUS ADVENTURE INTO HOW, WHAT, AND WHY WE TASTE

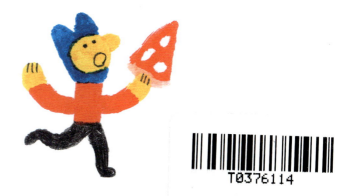

MICAELA CHIRIF · IGNACIO MEDINA · ANDREA ANTINORI

tra.publishing

Tongues are for speaking,

for eating ice cream,
for sticking out,
and, sometimes,
for licking your plate.

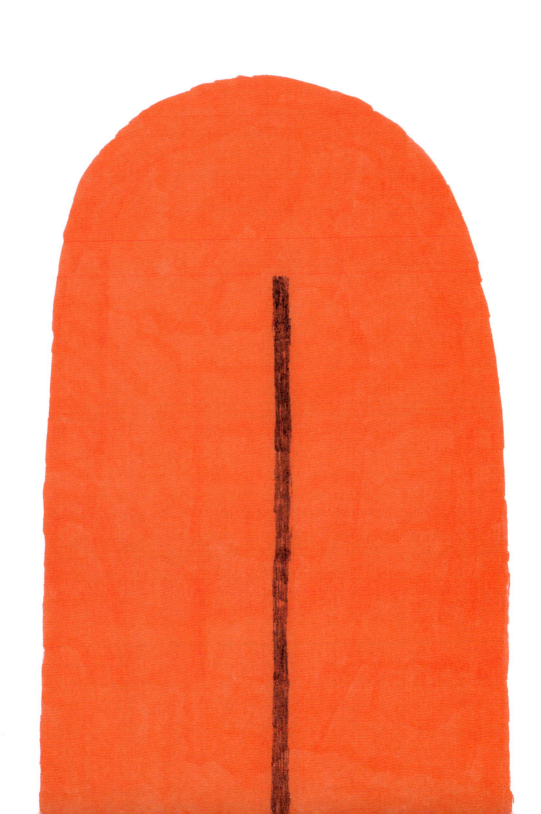

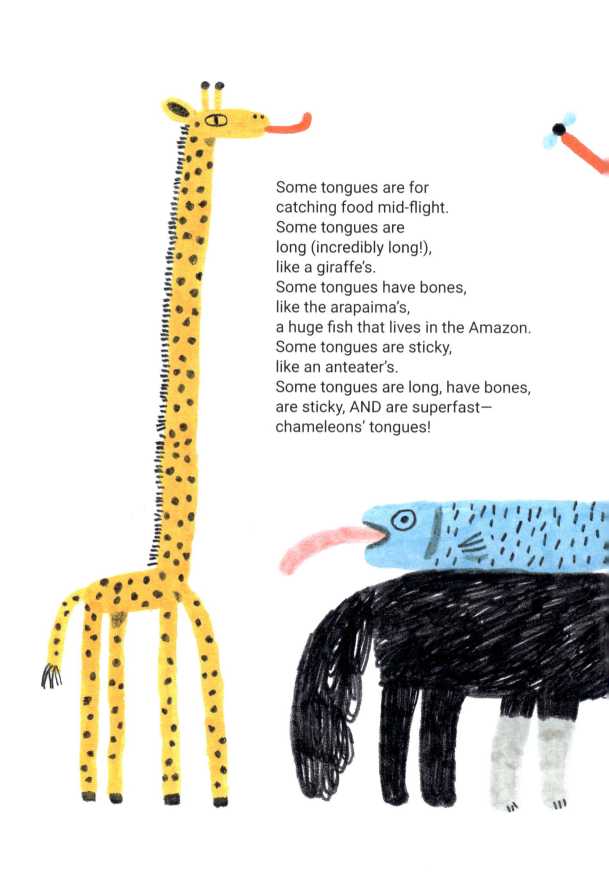

Some tongues are for catching food mid-flight. Some tongues are long (incredibly long!), like a giraffe's. Some tongues have bones, like the arapaima's, a huge fish that lives in the Amazon. Some tongues are sticky, like an anteater's. Some tongues are long, have bones, are sticky, AND are superfast— chameleons' tongues!

Anteaters can catch up to
thirty-five thousand ants with a single lick.

A chameleon's tongue can travel up
to twenty-six times the length of its own body
in just one second. It catches crickets,
flies, and grasshoppers before
they know what's hit them.

MY DOG STICKS OUT
HIS TONGUE
ALL THE TIME BECAUSE
HE'S HOT,
OR TO DRINK WATER.
I STICK MINE OUT
WHENEVER
I FEEL LIKE IT.

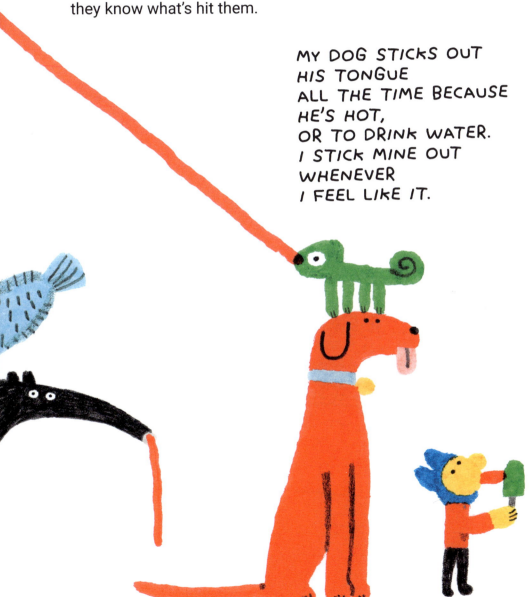

Tongues are for tasting the flavor of food.

If we didn't have any taste buds, everything would taste the same. In fact, it would be worse! Nothing would have any taste at all. We wouldn't be able to tell what we like from what we don't like. And we might also find it hard to tell what we can eat from what we can't eat, because a shoe would have the same flavor, or non-flavor, as a fried egg.

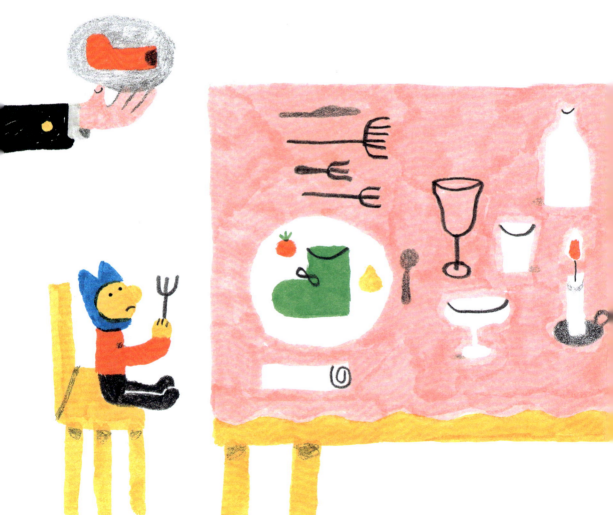

A human being's tongue has thousands of taste buds. If you stand in front of the mirror and stick out your tongue, you will see them.

A dog's tongue is smoother than ours because it has fewer taste buds. That means we are better than dogs at telling flavors apart.

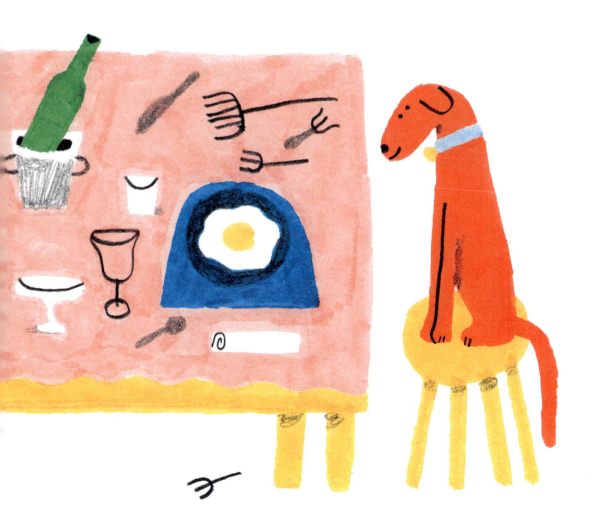

Flavors can be tasted all over our tongues,
but certain areas—the edges, the tip and the back—
are a little more sensitive.

Our palate and throat also have taste buds
that allow us to perceive the flavors of food.

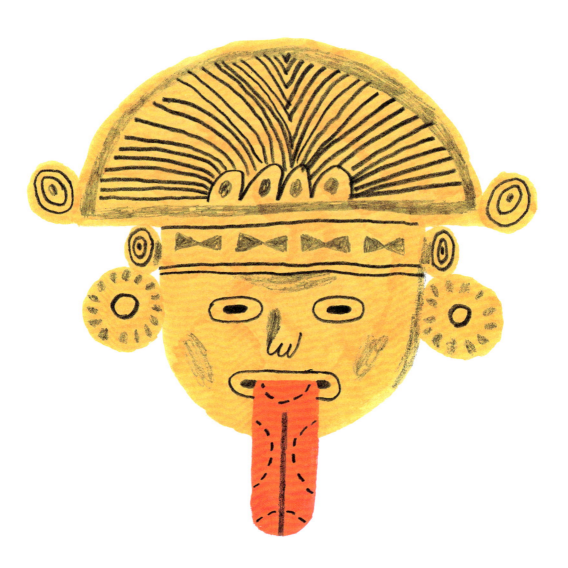

Our first food, milk, is sweet.

Our sweet tooth develops even before we are born. After only three months in the womb, a human fetus already has taste buds, and prefers sweet over bitter.

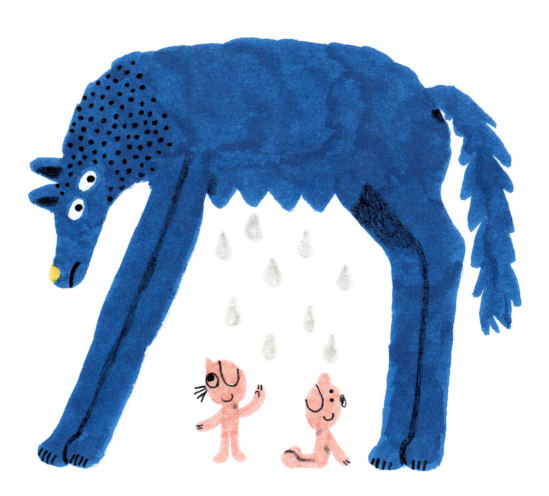

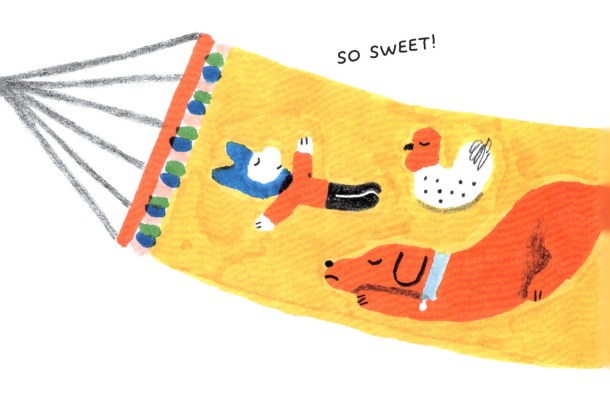

Sweetness is like gently swaying on a hammock until you fall asleep. It is like a love song, like a hug.

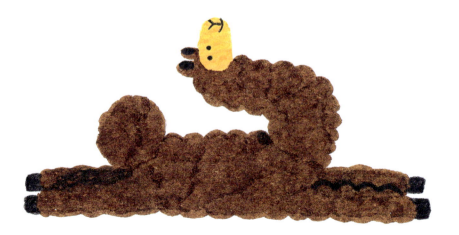

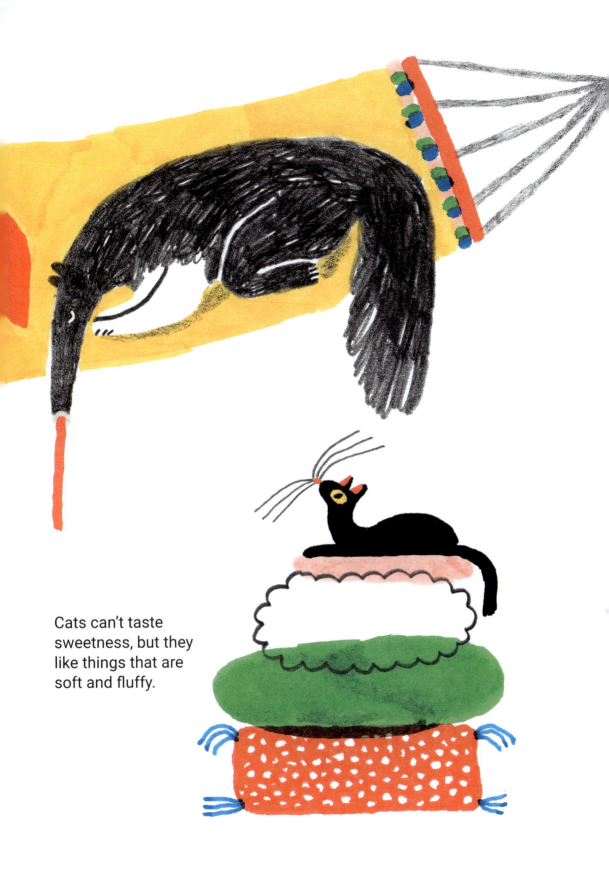

Cats can't taste sweetness, but they like things that are soft and fluffy.

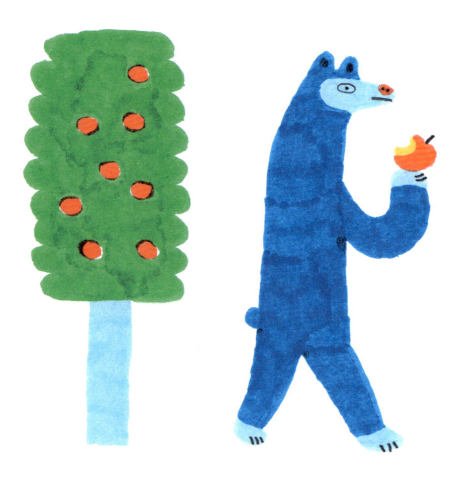

Some animals also have a sweet tooth, which can be useful for plants.

When seeds are not yet ready to reproduce, fruit tastes bitter or sour. That means animals don't eat it too early.

When they poop, animals expel the seeds of the fruit they have eaten. Those seeds grow into new plants, which produce more fruit. Then another animal comes along, and the cycle starts over.

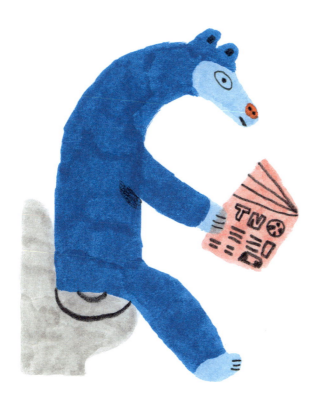
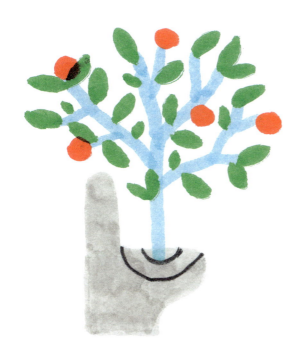
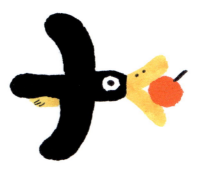

Sugar is sweet.

Candy is sweet.
Honey is sweet.
Apples, pears, bananas,
and mangoes are sweet.

Carrots and yams are sweet.
Onions can also be sweet,
even if they make you cry
when you chop them.

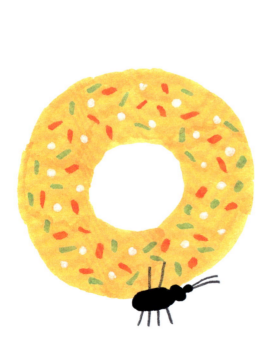
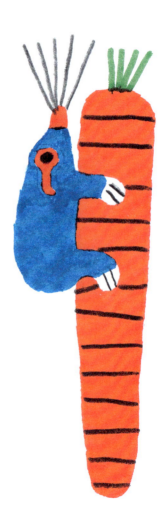

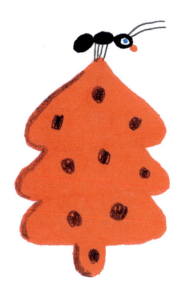
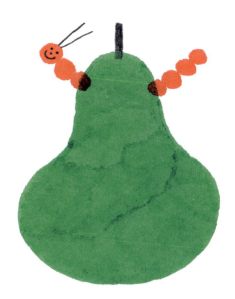
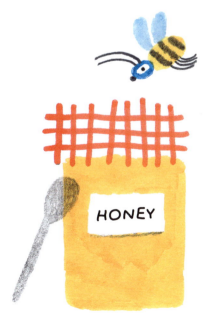
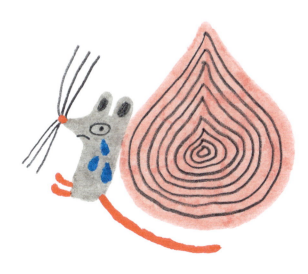

If you chop an onion, heat it up with a little oil over very low heat, and gently stir, you will notice that the water evaporates and the sugar it contains starts to concentrate. The onion becomes soft and sweet.

If you turn up the heat and keep stirring, the sugar caramelizes and the onion becomes darker.

If you turn up the heat even further, the sugar will burn, the onion stops being sweet, and turns bitter.

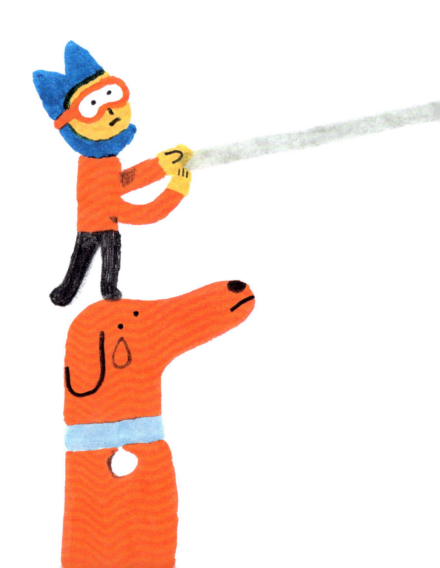

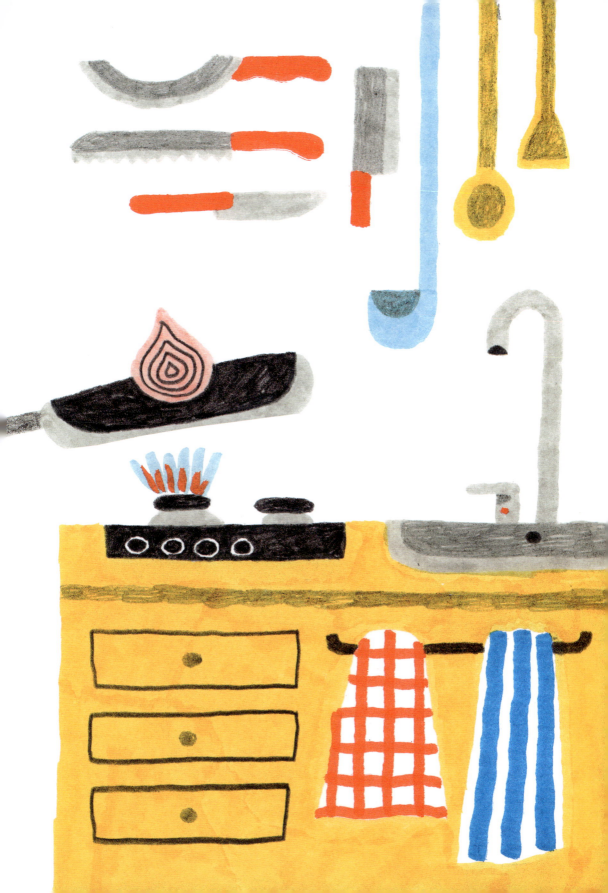

Many poisons are bitter. Our brain knows this, even though nobody has told us, so it rejects bitterness to protect us.

As we become older, we learn that bitter flavors are not always harmful, and we start to like them.

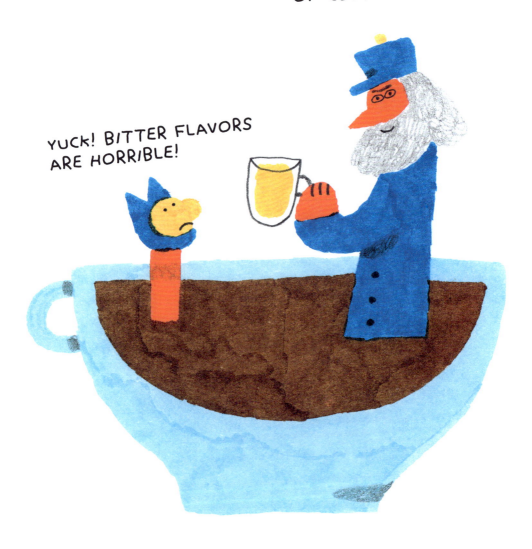

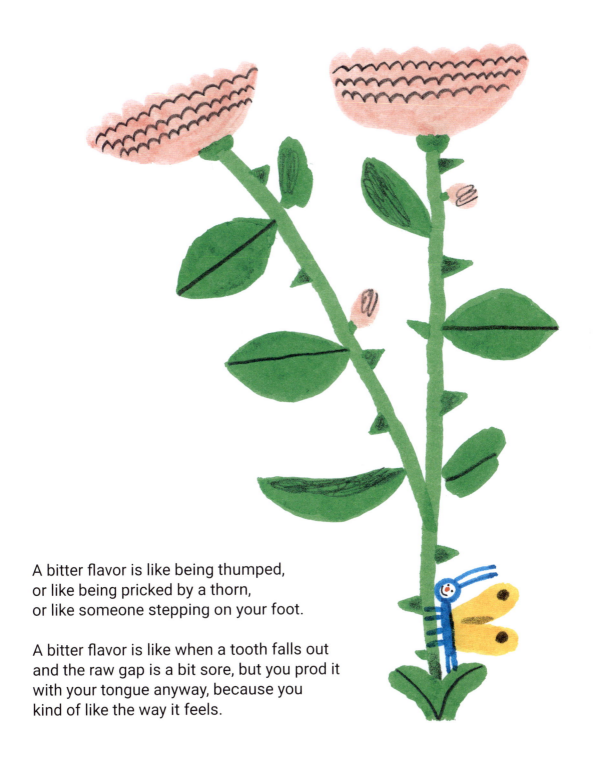

A bitter flavor is like being thumped,
or like being pricked by a thorn,
or like someone stepping on your foot.

A bitter flavor is like when a tooth falls out
and the raw gap is a bit sore, but you prod it
with your tongue anyway, because you
kind of like the way it feels.

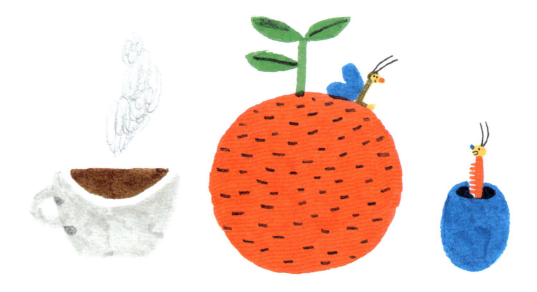
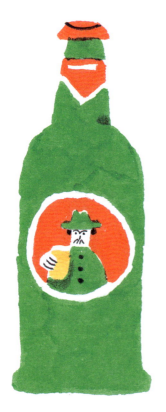

Coffee and beer are bitter.
Olives and orange peel are bitter.

Chocolate is also bitter.

CHOCOLATE???

Chocolate is sweet!

That is why
we eat chocolate cake
at birthday parties,
and chocolate ice cream
at ice cream parlors,
and chocolate cookies
at Grandma's.

Chocolate is made from cacao. Cacao beans are sweet, sour, and only a tiny bit bitter, but they become more bitter when you dry them and roast them to make chocolate.

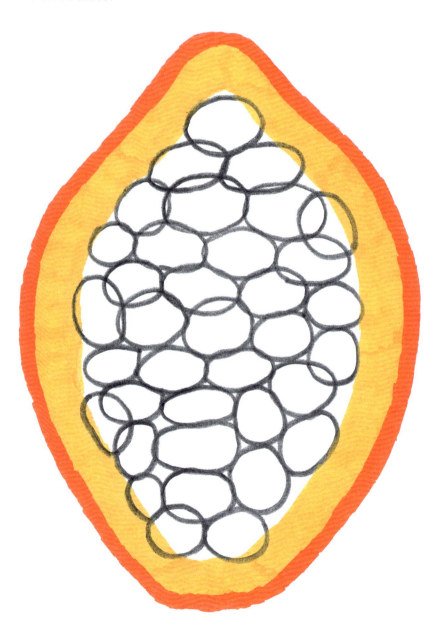

So, if you don't add any sugar,

chocolate is bitter.

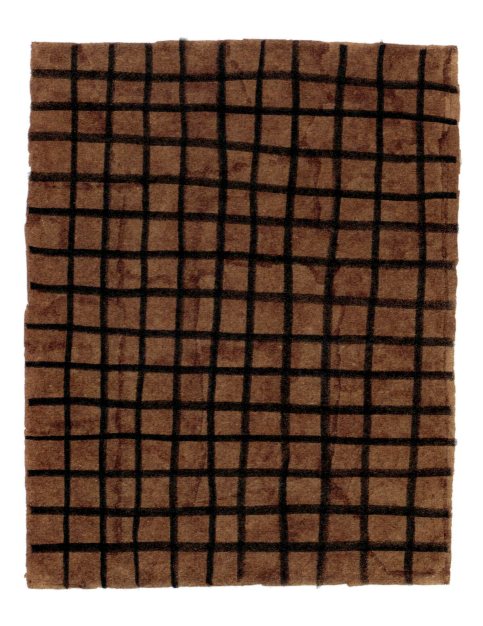

Cacao is native to the Amazon region, but chocolate was first created in what is now Mexico. It was called *xocolatl* and it was made into a bitter, spicy drink.

In the 16th century, the Spaniards replaced the spiciness of *xocolatl* with sugar. So, it became a little bit bitter and a little bit sweet.

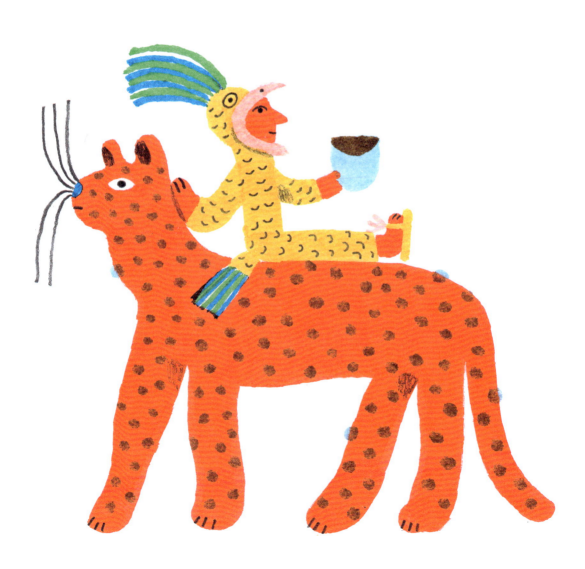

At the end of the 19th century,
the Swiss added some milk to the sugar.
This is how the flavor of chocolate
became sweeter and less bitter.
Since then, people have added hazelnuts,
raisins, walnuts, and even tomato,
ants, and bacon!

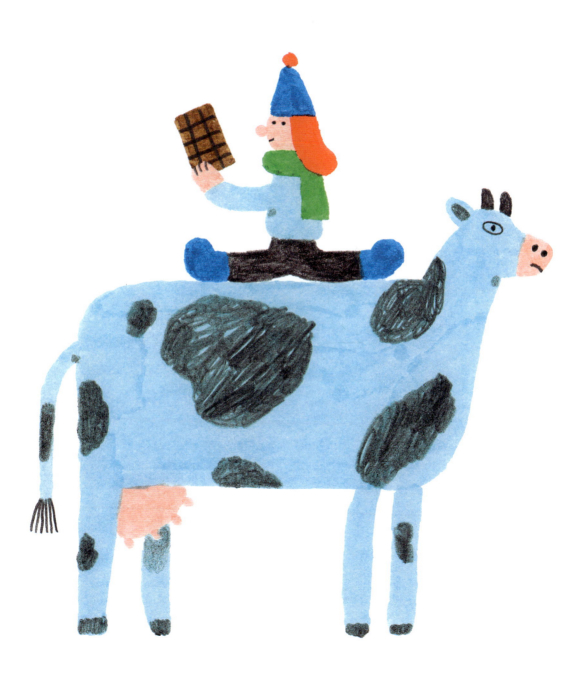

WELL, I DON'T WANT
ANY ANTS IN MY CHOCOLATE!
I LIKE MY CHOCOLATE SWEET
AND MELTED.
I LIKE IT SO MUCH THAT
I WOULD LOVE TO BE A FISH
AND SPEND MY DAYS SWIMMING
IN A SEA OF CHOCOLATE.

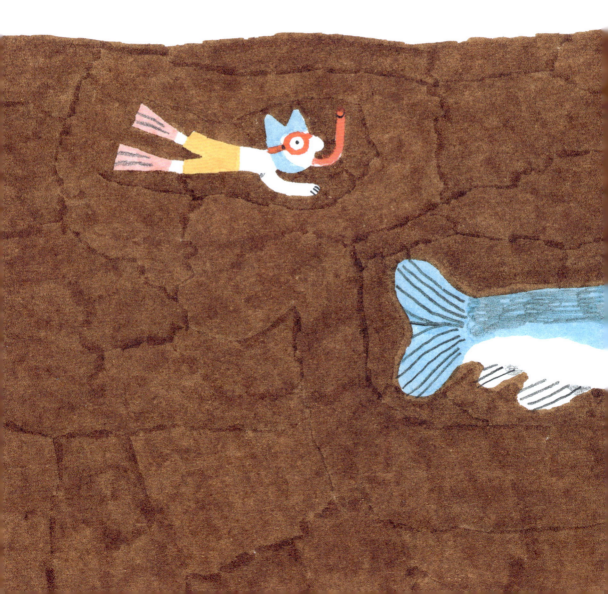

If you swam in chocolate
you might want to be a catfish.

Catfish have many more taste
buds than humans. And they have
them all over their body!

Chickens, however, only have
24 taste buds and can't swim at all.

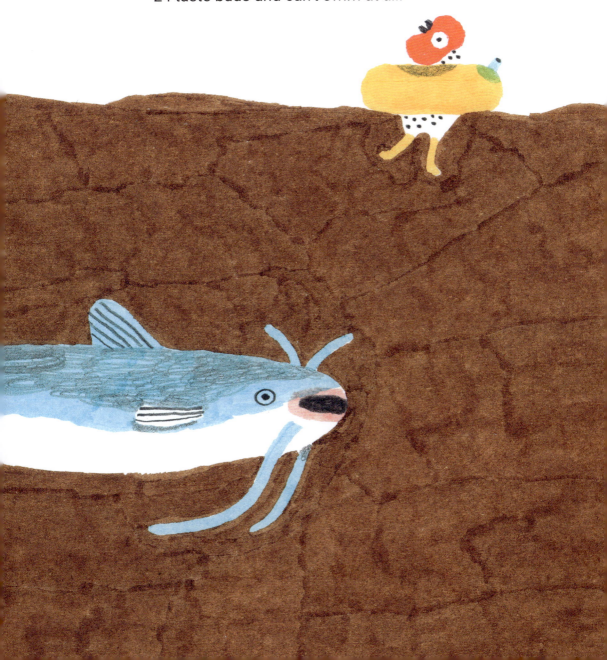

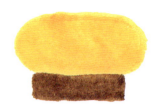

Chocolate can be
sweet or bitter,
or sweet and bitter,
or spicy,
or sour,
or even salty.
But it always smells like chocolate.

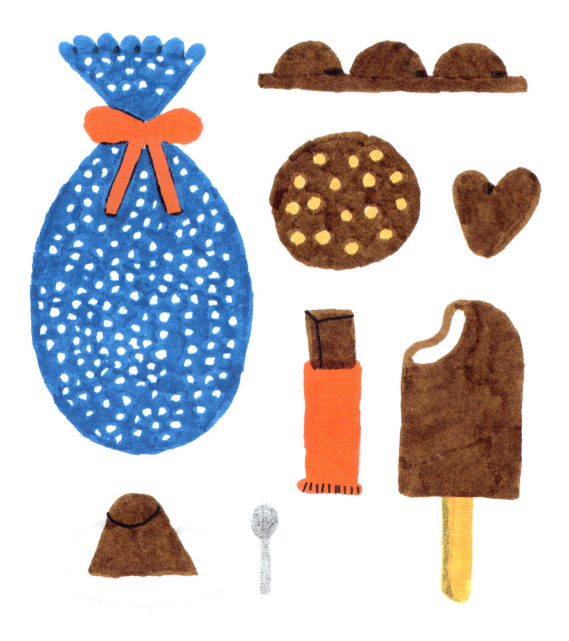

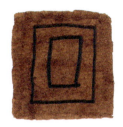
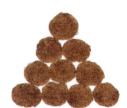

Cover your nose and eat some chocolate.

It tastes sweet and possibly a little bitter, but if it doesn't smell like chocolate, then it won't taste like chocolate. More than half of what we think of as taste is, in fact, smell.

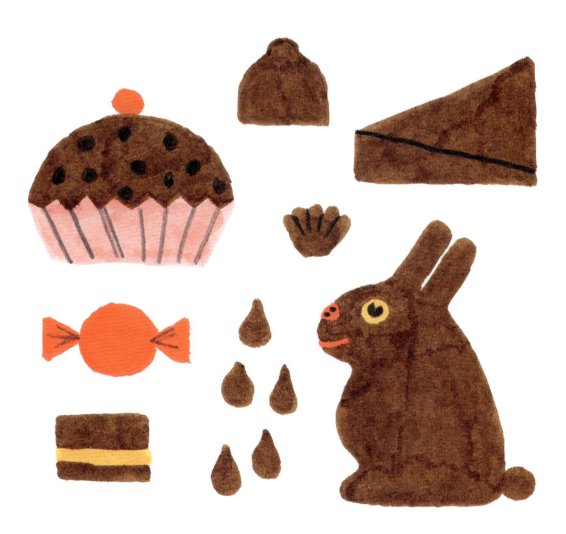

When we chew our food, its smell travels up to our noses. That is why we confuse smell with taste.

If you cover your nose, you stop the air from circulating upwards from your mouth to your nose, and your olfactory (or scent) cells no longer perceive the smell of what you are eating. That is why when you have a cold, you can't taste your food as much, because you can't smell it properly!

Many popsicles, candies, chewing gums, or yogurts don't taste like strawberry, mango, or banana. Most of them don't even contain any real strawberry or mango or banana. But they smell like strawberry, mango, and banana because they have added aromas that remind us of the smell of those fruits.

These aromas, often called flavorings, makes us think we are eating strawberries or mangoes or bananas, even if we are only smelling them.

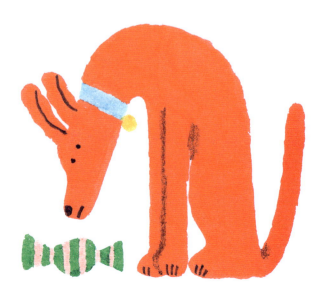

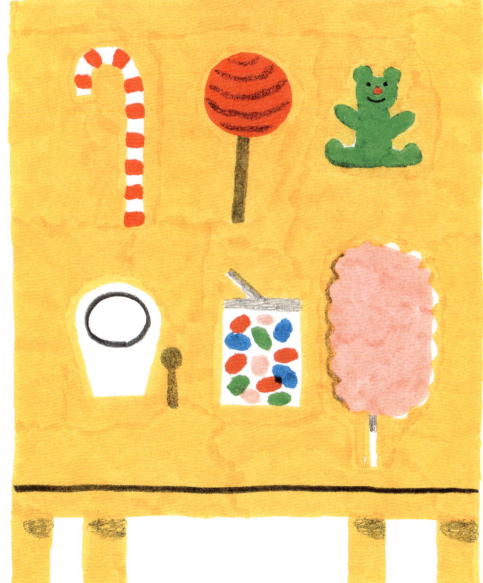

Spices are smells.

Some are flowers, like saffron;
others are herbs, like parsley,
cilantro, mint, or oregano;
others are bark, like cinnamon;
or seeds, like pepper or mustard;
or roots, like ginger.

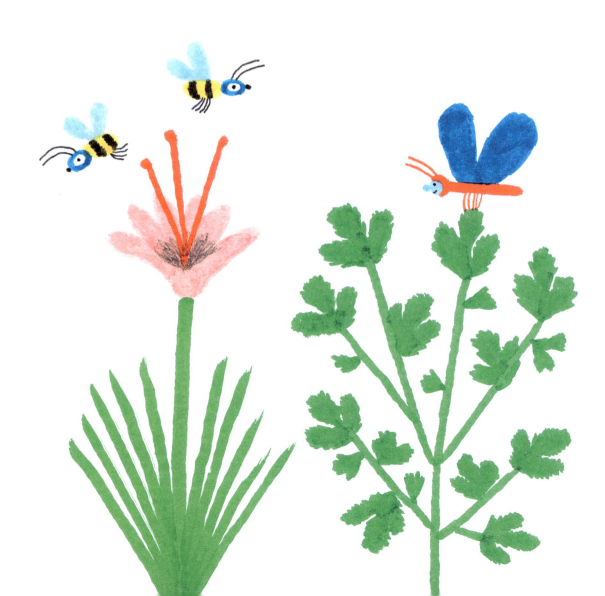

Sometimes we use them fresh;
other times, they are dry.

They can be whole, chopped, or ground.
Some are spicy, others are sour, sweet, or bitter,
but they are all used to make dishes more flavorful with
their aromas. (Sometimes, they are useful for covering
up the smell of produce that isn't very fresh.)

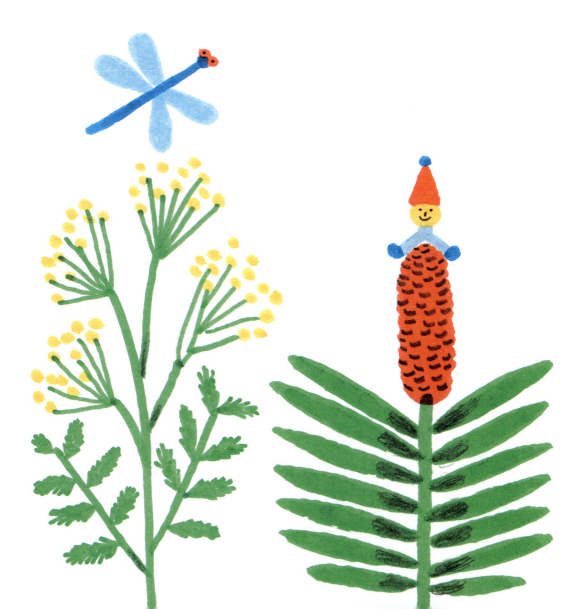

Many animals have a better sense of smell than we do,

like dogs, guinea pigs, cows, and horses.

Being so good at smelling helps them find food and detect the presence of predators that might otherwise gobble them up.

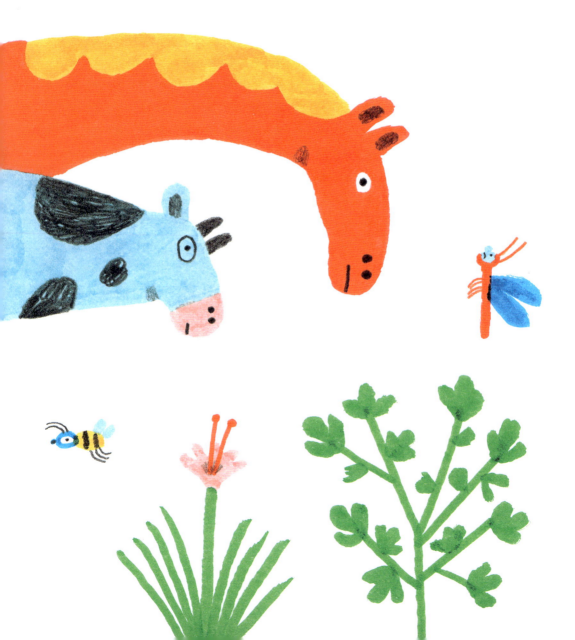

No one has a better sense
of smell than the African elephant,
which can make out smells from
a distance of six miles.

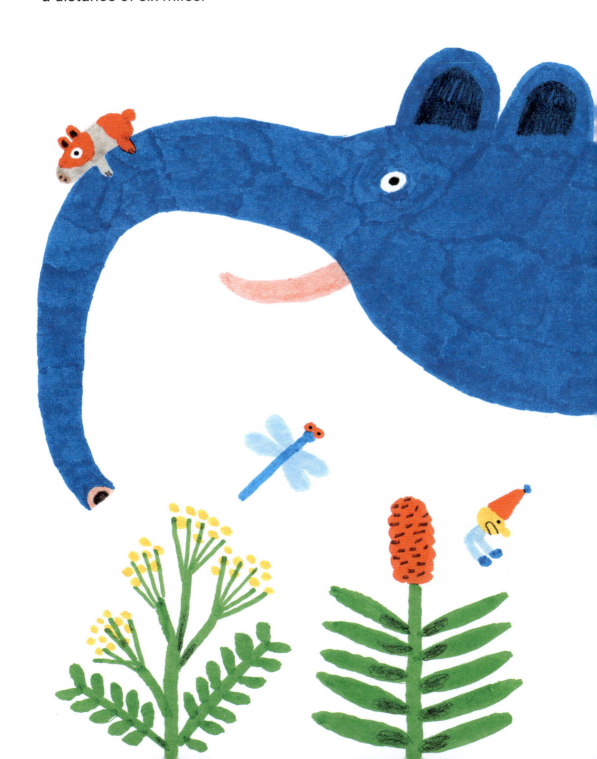

We taste flavors with our tongue and our
nose, but also, a little bit, with our eyes.

If you see an apple,
you expect it to taste like apple,
not sausage or soup.

If you see a bowl of soup,
you expect it to taste like soup,
not chewing gum.

If you see a red candy,
you expect it to taste like cherry
or strawberry, but not lemon.

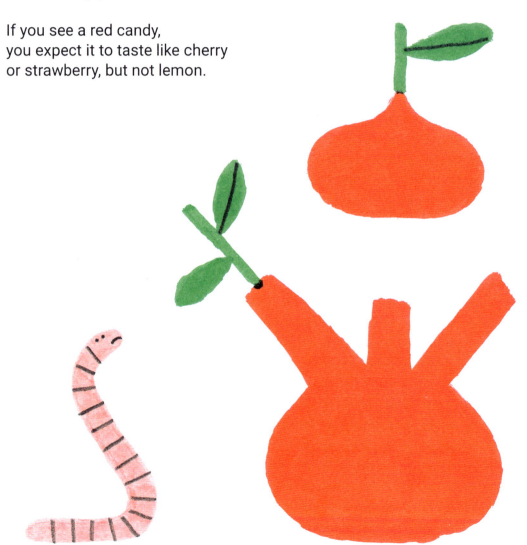

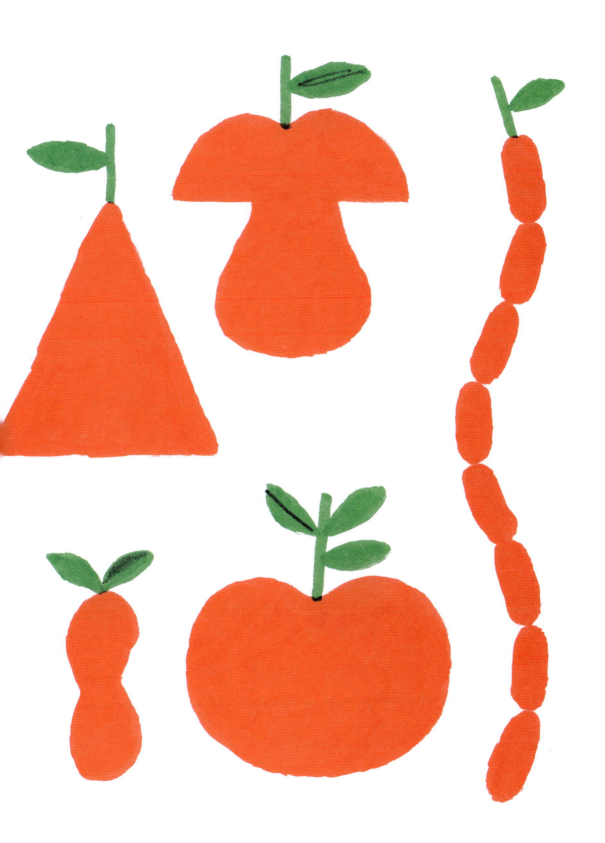

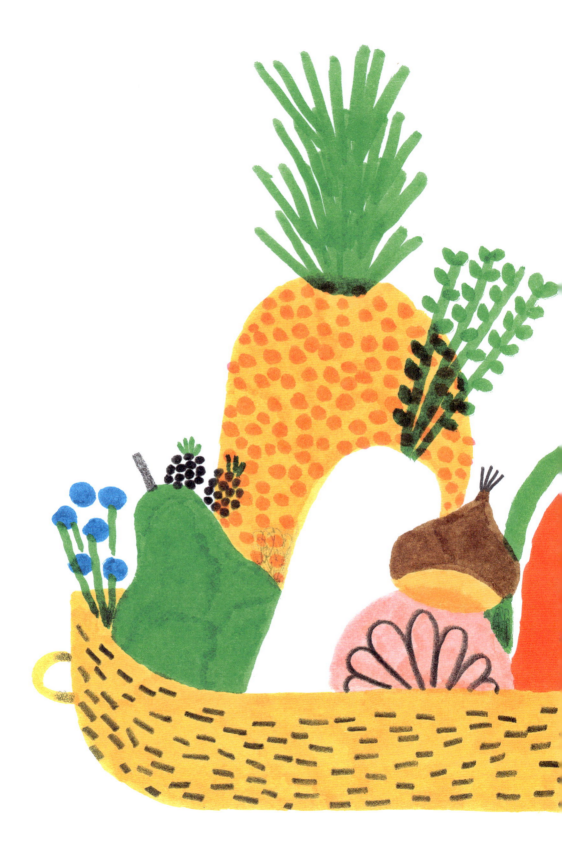

There are red foods,
white foods,
green foods,
and yellow foods.
There are brown foods,
like chestnuts.
There are purple foods,
like blueberries and plums.
There are black foods,
like squid ink.
There are very few blue foods.

Blue food is rare.
The only genuinely blue
fruit is the blue quandong,
which grows in Australia.

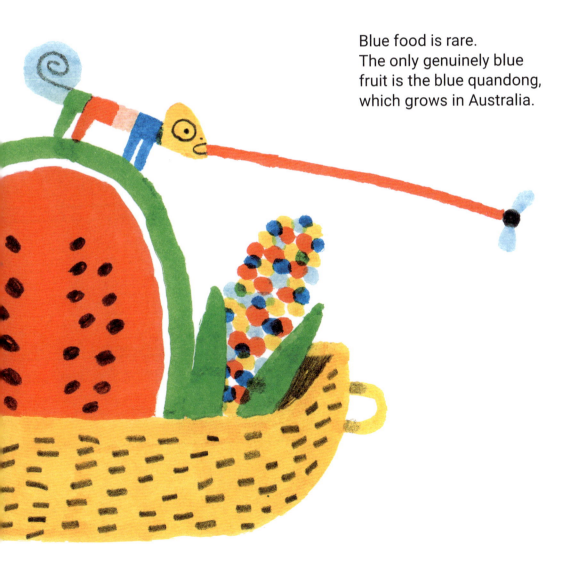

Strawberries are red.
Red doesn't taste like anything.

What do you mean?!
Red tastes like strawberry.

And what does a strawberry taste like?
It's juicy like a melon.

And what does a melon taste like?
It's soft like a peach.

And what does a peach taste like?
It's sweet like a fig.

And what does a fig taste like?
It's delicious like a strawberry.

Watermelon is red but does
not taste like strawberry.

Grapes are green but do not
 taste like lettuce.

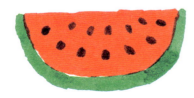

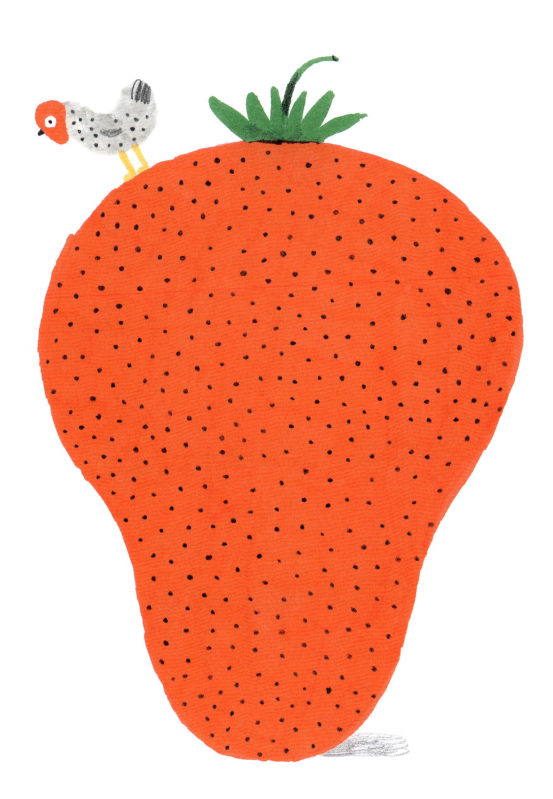

Squeeze a lemon into your mouth.

That is what sour tastes like.

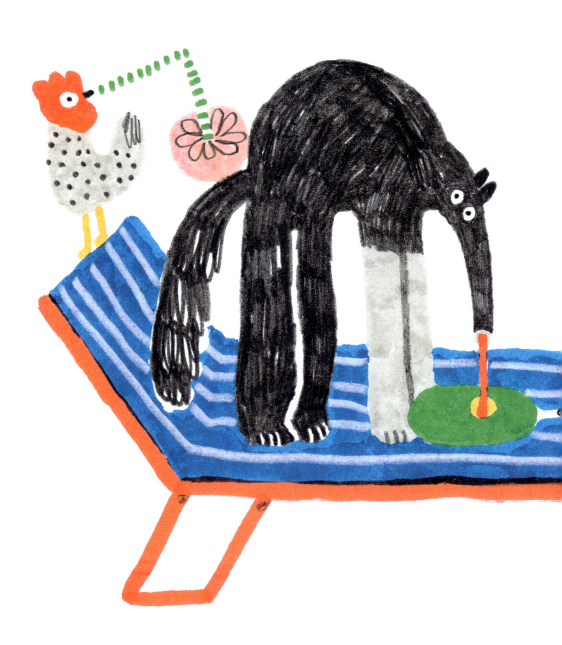

When you think of something sour,
like a lemon,
a grapefruit,
a passion fruit,
a green mango,
or a spoonful of vinegar,
your mouth fills up with saliva.

Sour flavors, like bitter flavors, make alarm bells
go off in our brains, because some
sour substances are not good for our bodies.
We produce saliva to help dissolve
the sourness.

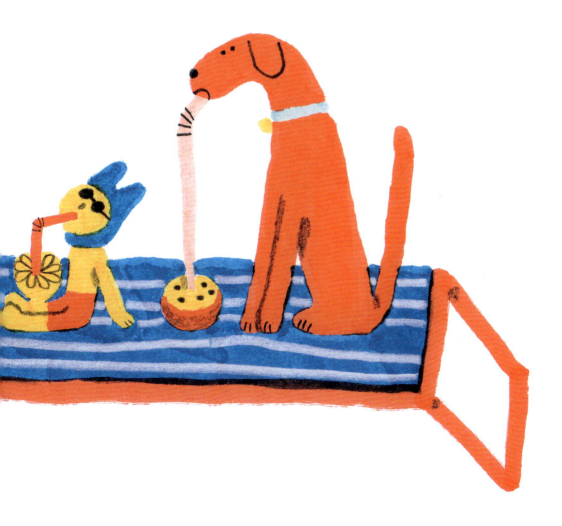

If we could touch sourness, it might be covered in small spikes or it might crackle with electricity.

I LIKE SOUR FOOD. IT MAKES ME FEEL AWAKE, LIKE COLD RAIN IS FALLING ON MY FACE AND DOWN THE INSIDE OF MY BACK.

IT MAKES ME FEEL LIKE EYES HAVE SUDDENLY OPENED UP ALL OVER MY BODY.

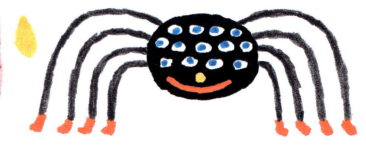

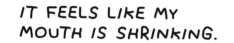
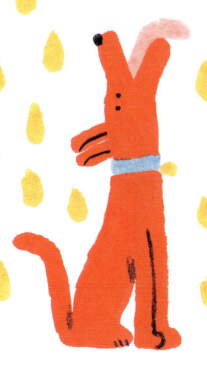
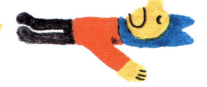

Everything has a flavor,
even water.
Because rainwater
is different from tap water,
is different from river water,
is different from hose water,
is different from seawater.
Seawater is salty.

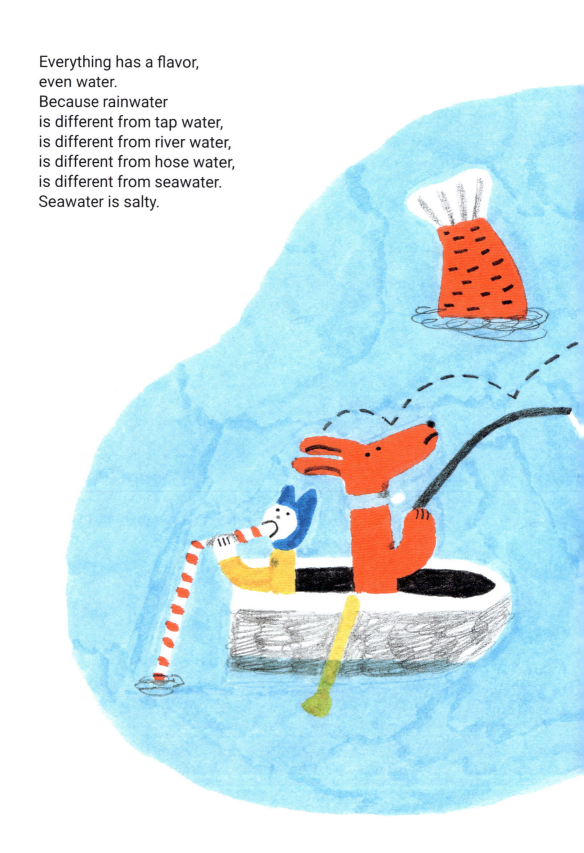

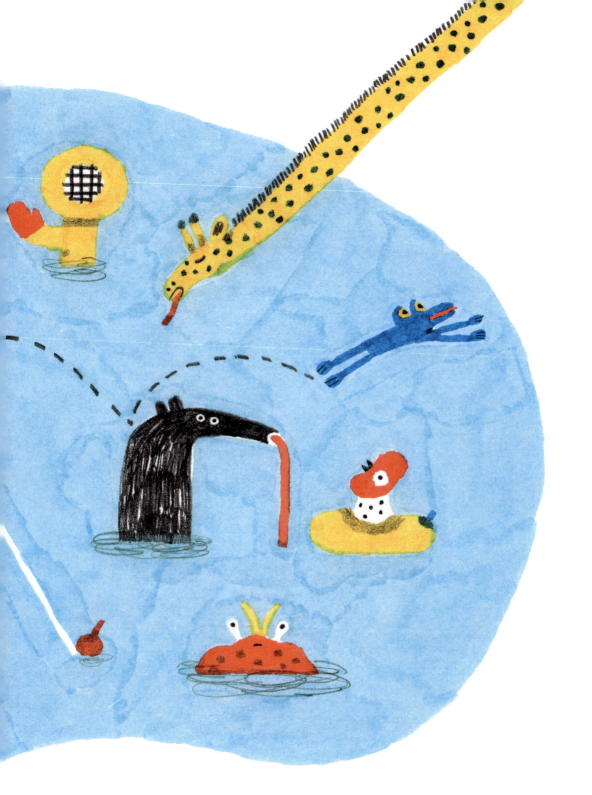

People also have a flavor.
If you jump and play a lot, and then
lick your arm, you will notice that
your skin has a salty flavor from
the sweat.

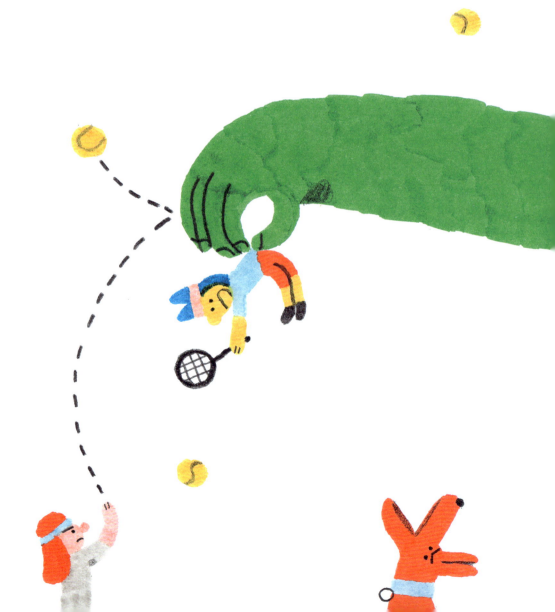

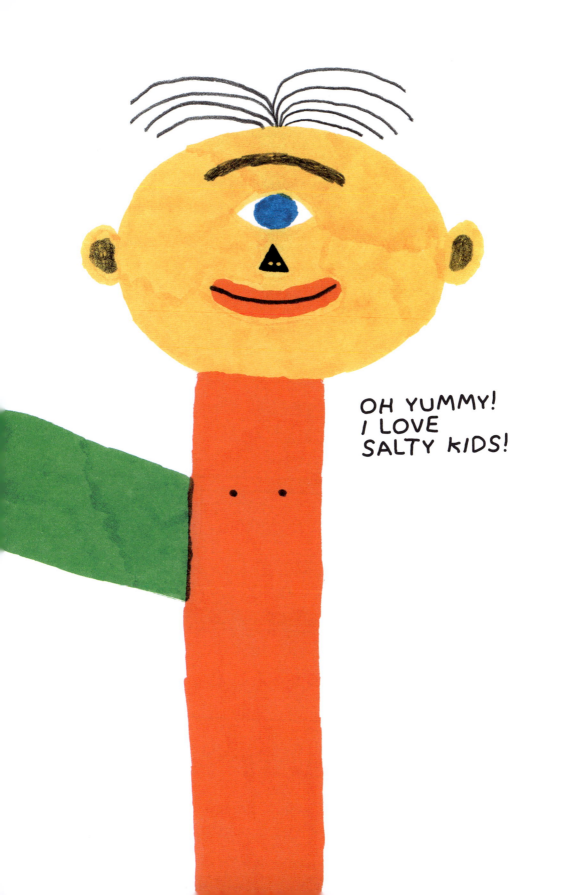

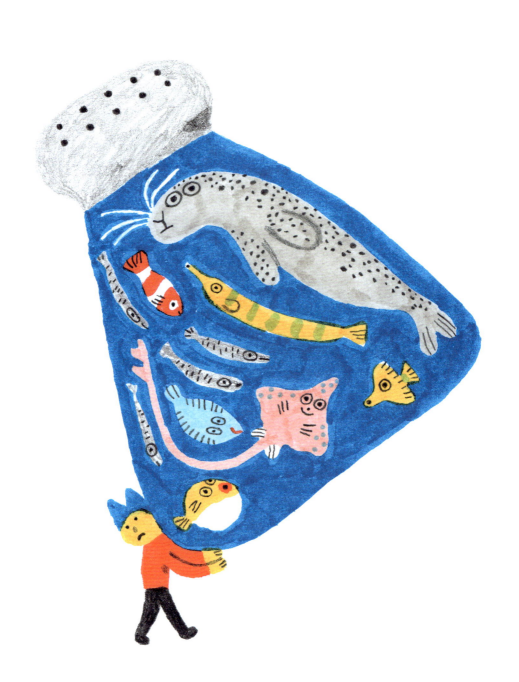

The salt we use at the table
can come from the sea
or from the earth.

Salt makes food salty.

Dogs cannot taste salt very well.
That is why they sometimes drink
seawater and then get a tummy ache.

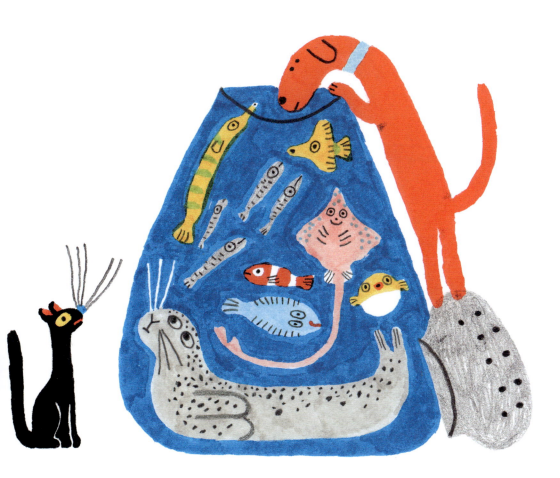

Aside from sweet, salty, sour, and bitter, there is another flavor called umami.

Umami means 'tasty' in Japanese.

This flavor was first identified a little more than a hundred years ago.

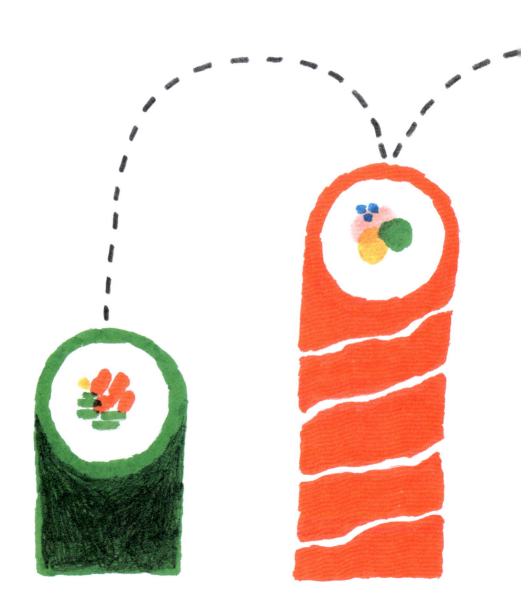

Umami is salty, but not only salty.
It's bitter, but not only bitter.
It's sour, but not only sour.
It's a kind of mix of flavors.

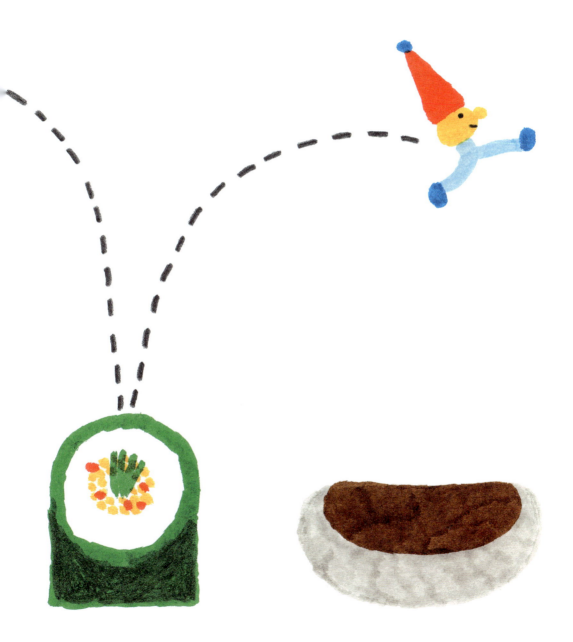

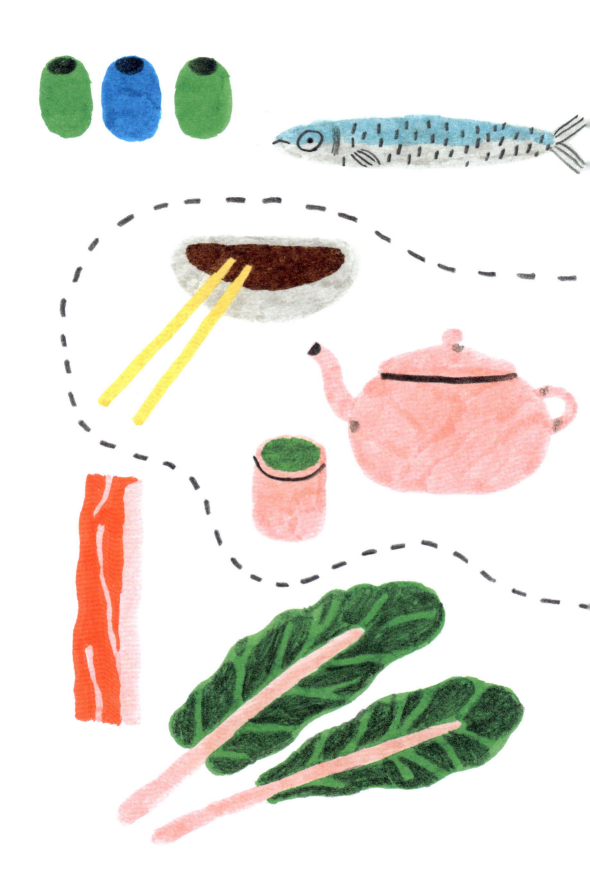

Glutamate, a substance that can be found in many foods, is what gives us the umami flavor.

If you discover what the flavors of these foods have in common, you will have discovered umami.

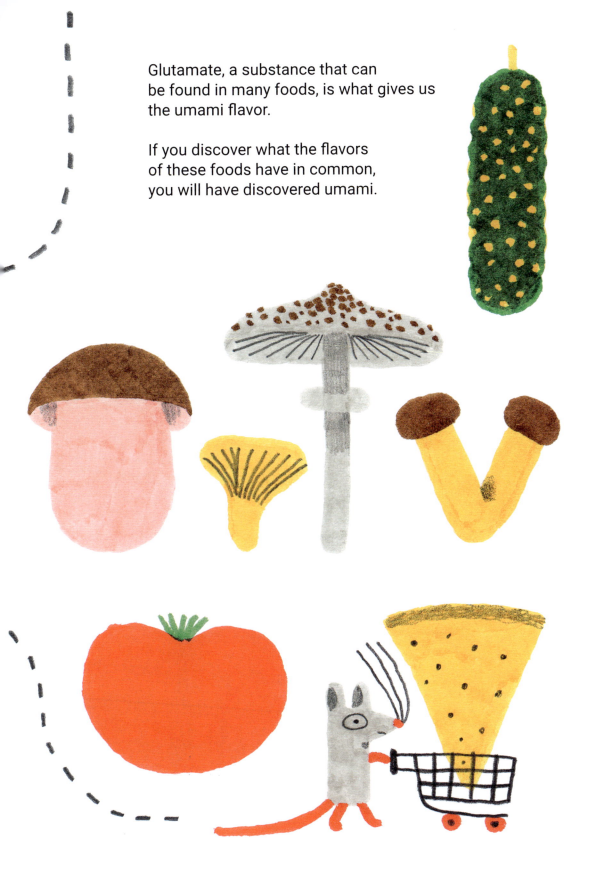

Sweet is a flavor,
bitter is a flavor,
sour is a flavor,
salty is a flavor,
umami is a flavor.

Spiciness is not exactly a flavor. It is heat.

It is a kind of heat that some people really like and others don't like at all.

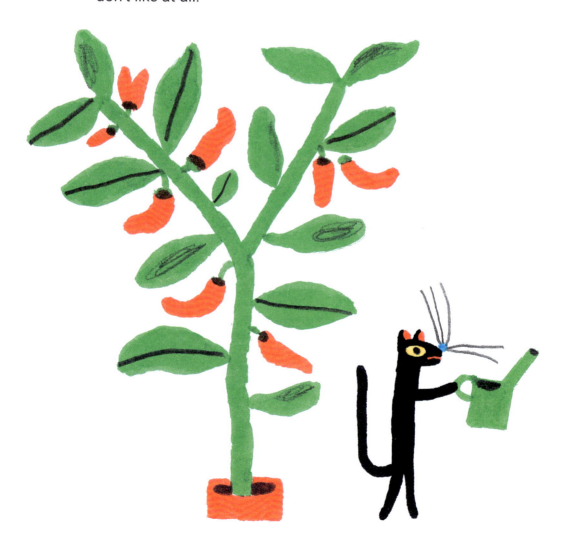

When we eat spicy food, our brain thinks we are burning. To fight the burning feeling, it releases substances called endorphins, which make us feel good. This makes us feel like eating more spicy food, so we can release more endorphins.

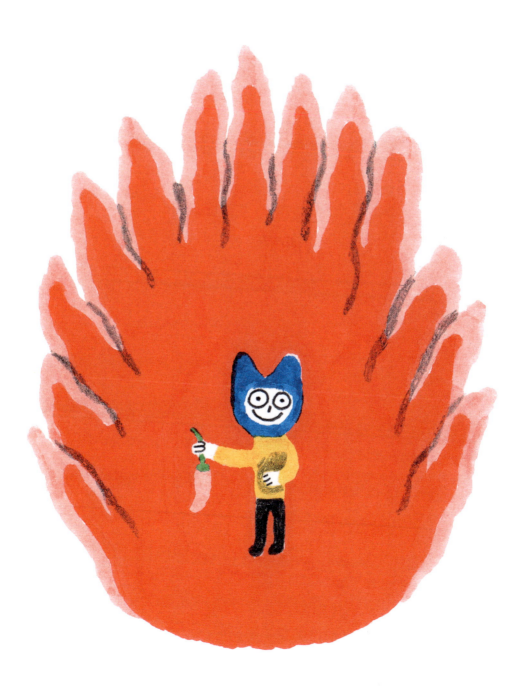

Eating spicy food is like going on a rollercoaster.

You scream a lot on the way up,
and then you feel happy going back down.

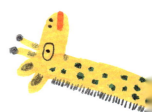

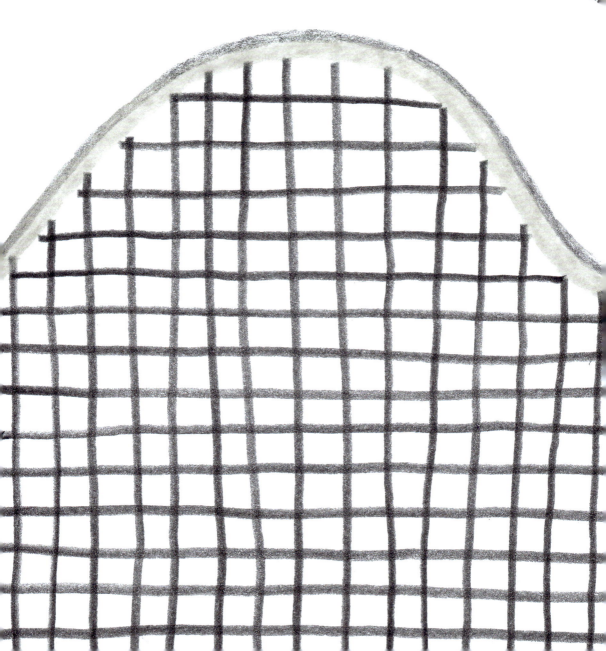

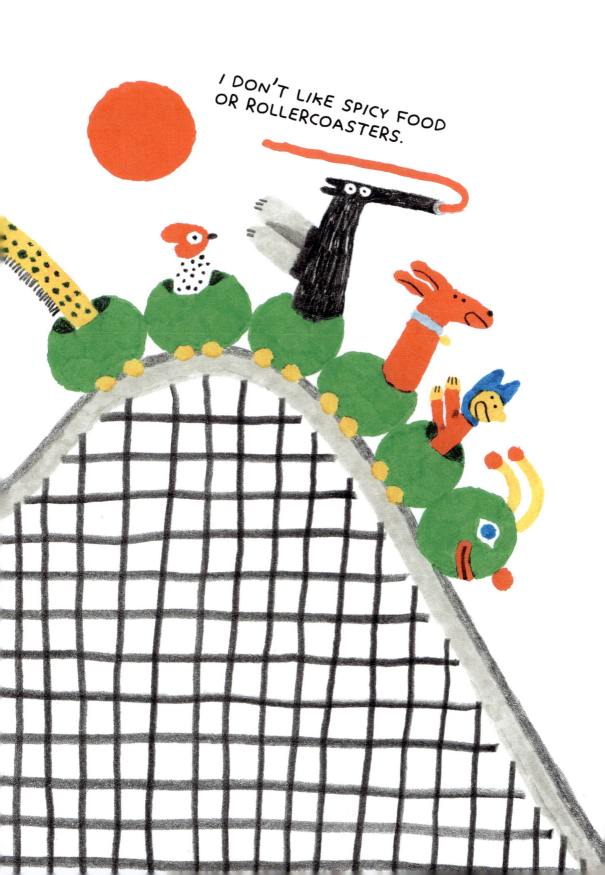

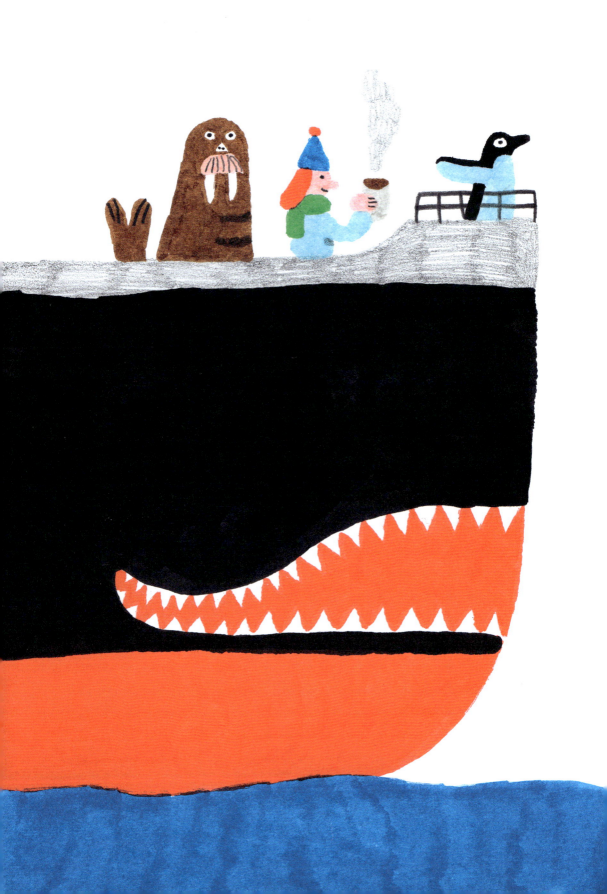

This isn't spicy, but it burns.

Food is more flavorful when eaten warm, but if you eat it when it's too hot you will burn your tongue, and your taste buds won't be able to taste flavors so well.

Hot and cold are not flavors, but it is different to eat food when it is cold or hot. We like ice cream to be cold and stew to be hot.

Sometimes we enjoy the temperature of food even more than its flavor. That's why we drink water with ice when we are hot, and hot chocolate when we are cold.

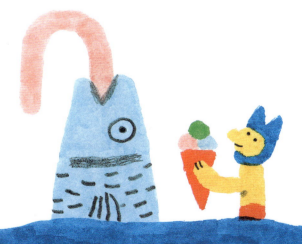

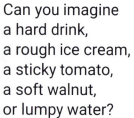

Can you imagine
a hard drink,
a rough ice cream,
a sticky tomato,
a soft walnut,
or lumpy water?

As well as flavors and temperatures,

our mouths feel textures.

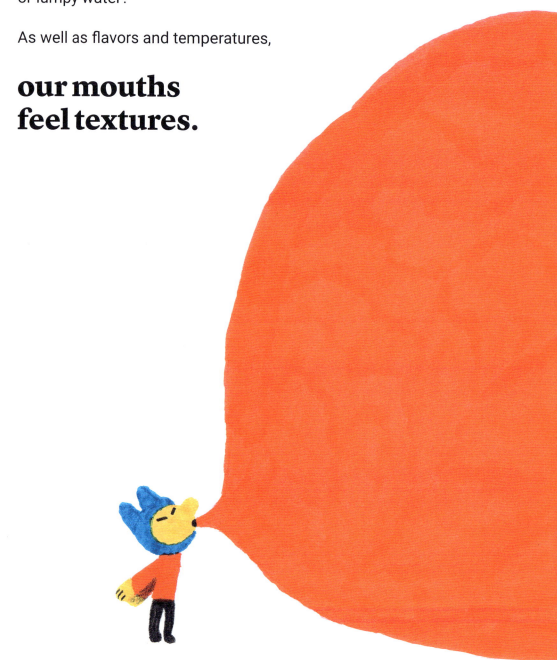

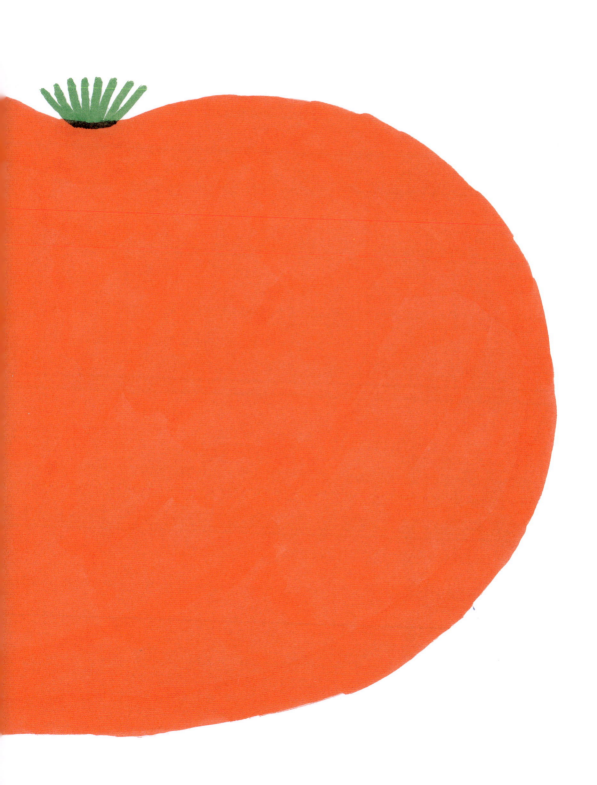

Having something sweet and sticky is not
the same as having something sweet and hard,
or sweet and soft, or sweet and rough.

Ice cream is cold, but it is also soft.
Soup is warm and liquid,
candy is sometimes hard,
melted cheese is gooey,
and green bananas are astringent.

Astringent?
Yes, it's a mix of rough and dry.

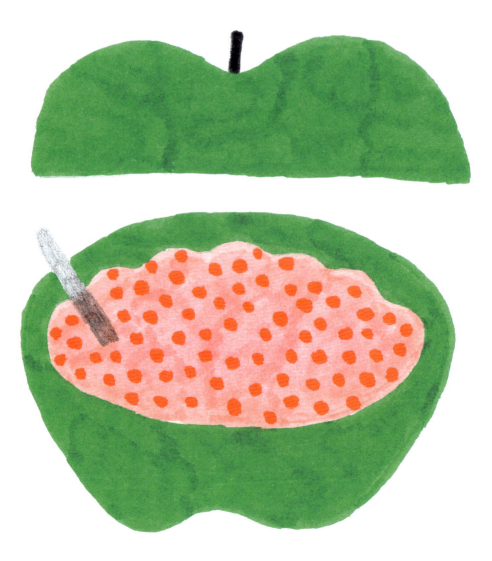

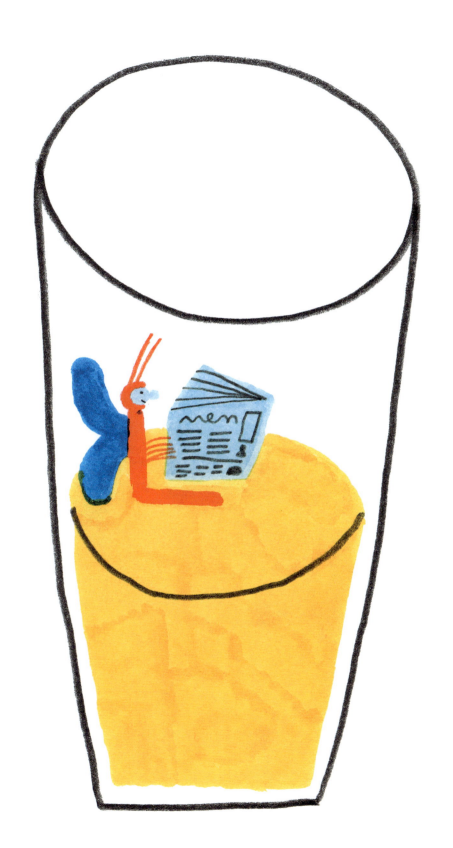

If you wait too long to eat an ice cream,
it warms up and melts.

If you age a piece of cheese,
its taste becomes stronger.

The flavor of some foods
changes over time.

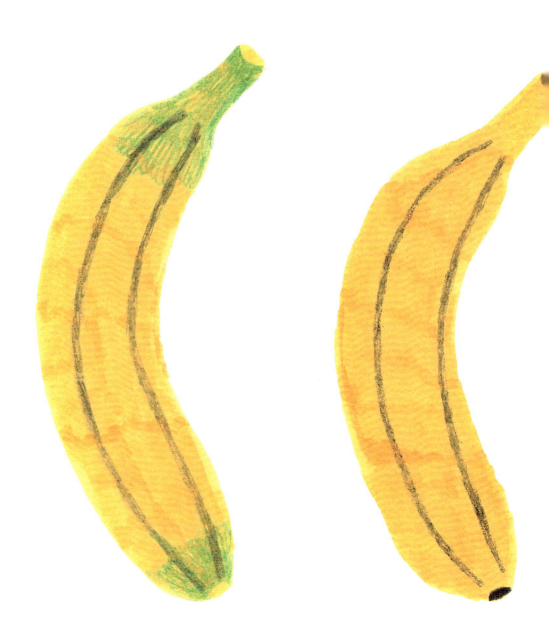

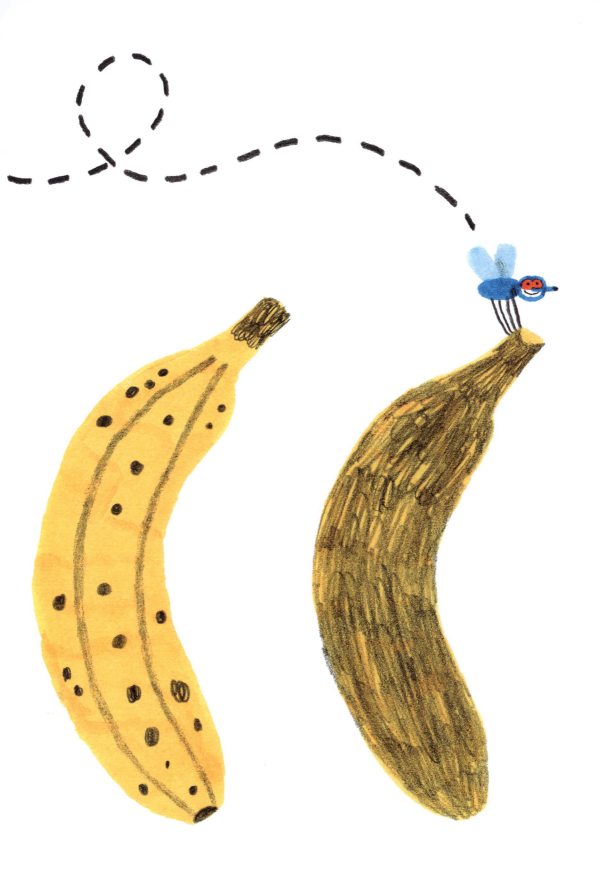

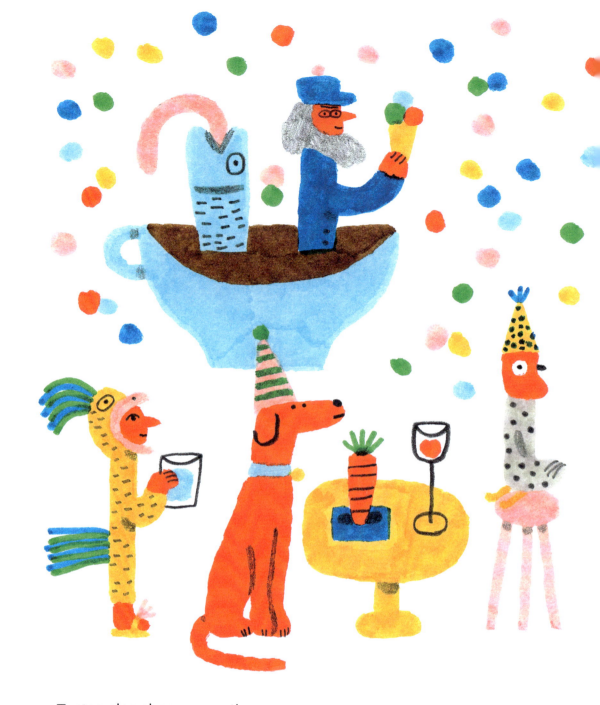

Tastes also change over time,
and from one person to another.

We are all different, and we like different things.

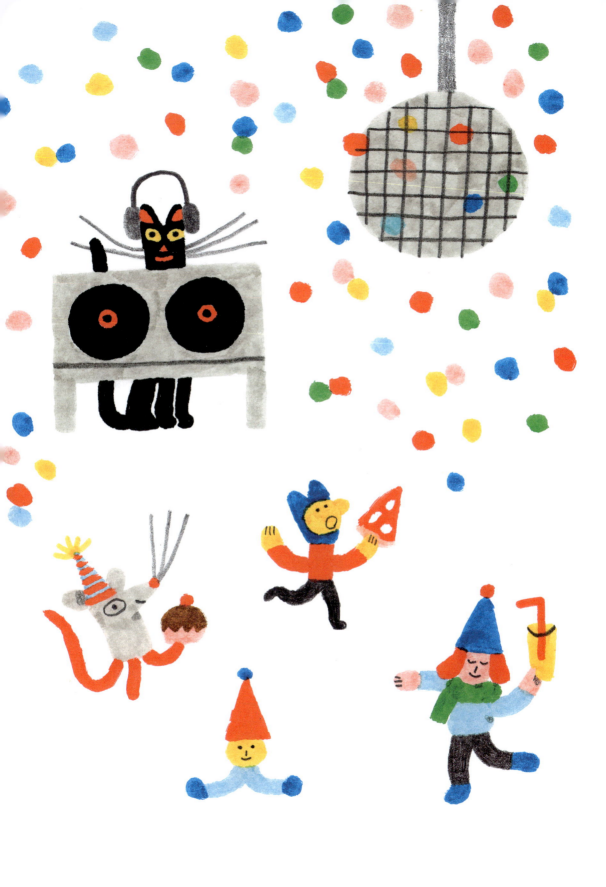

Would it possible to make
a hamburger that tastes like strawberry?

Would all colors of the rainbow
have the same flavor?

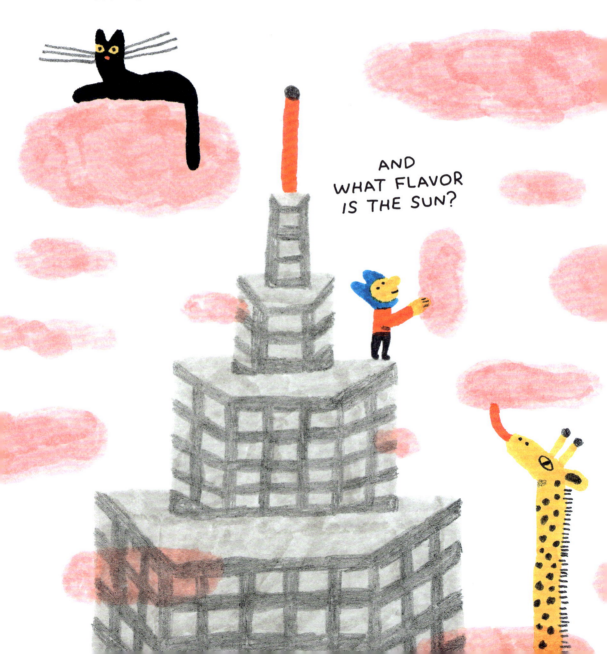

If sweet were a color, what would it be?
If we could touch salty, perhaps it would feel like sand, and sour would feel like a river.

It would be wonderful to create an ice cream that changes its flavor after each lick.

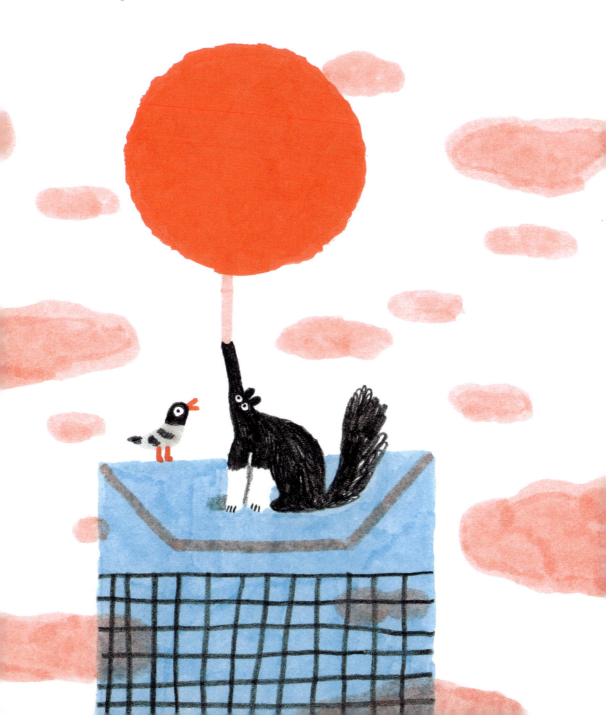

Sometimes flavor does not only
depend on the food.

Eating in good company
is not the same as eating alone;
eating in a happy mood is not the same
as eating when we are angry;
eating when we are hungry is not the same
as eating with no appetite;
eating one pie is not the same
as eating three;
eating in the morning is not the
same as eating at night;
eating while we are awake
is not the same as...

eating while we are asleep?

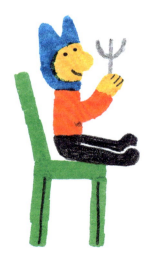
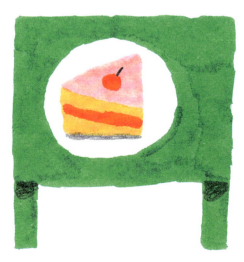

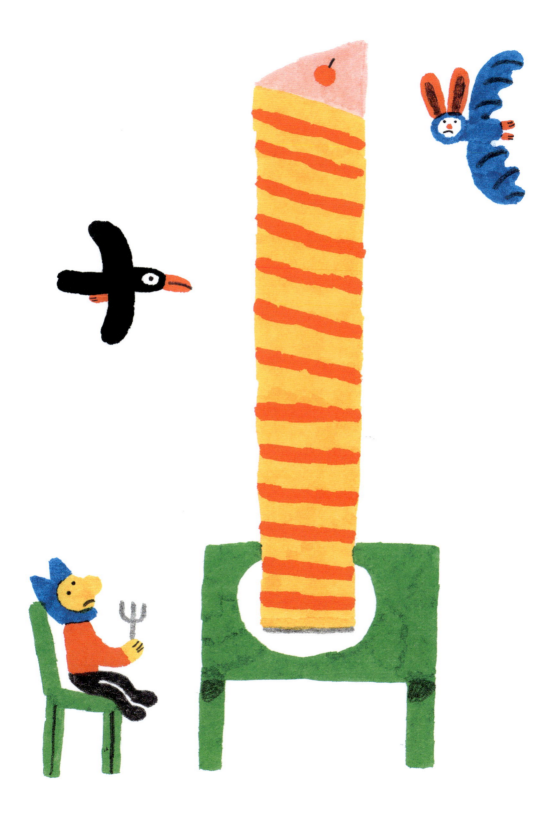

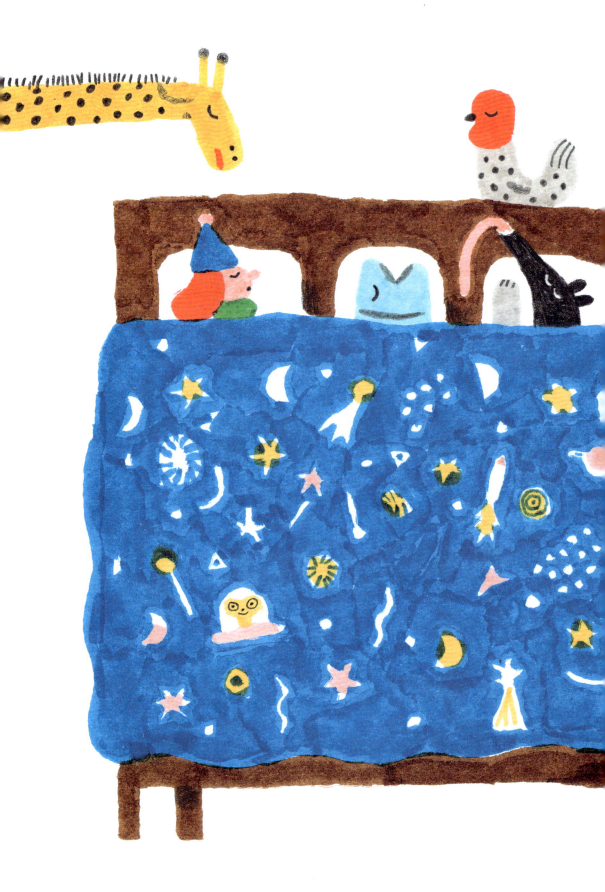

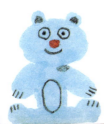

We can't eat while we are asleep!

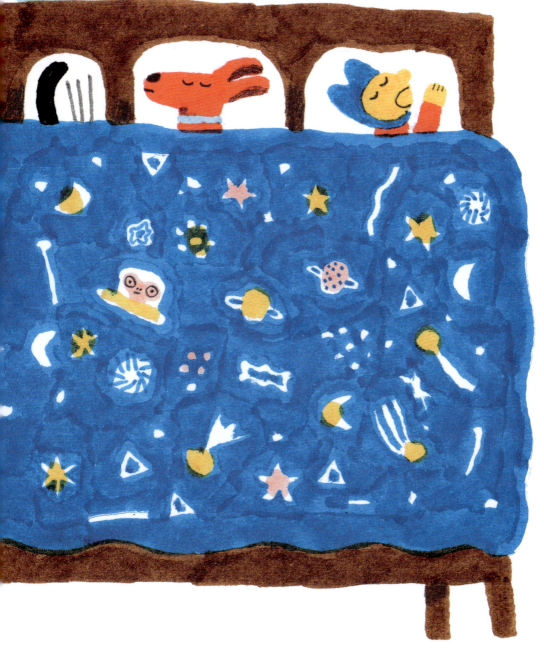

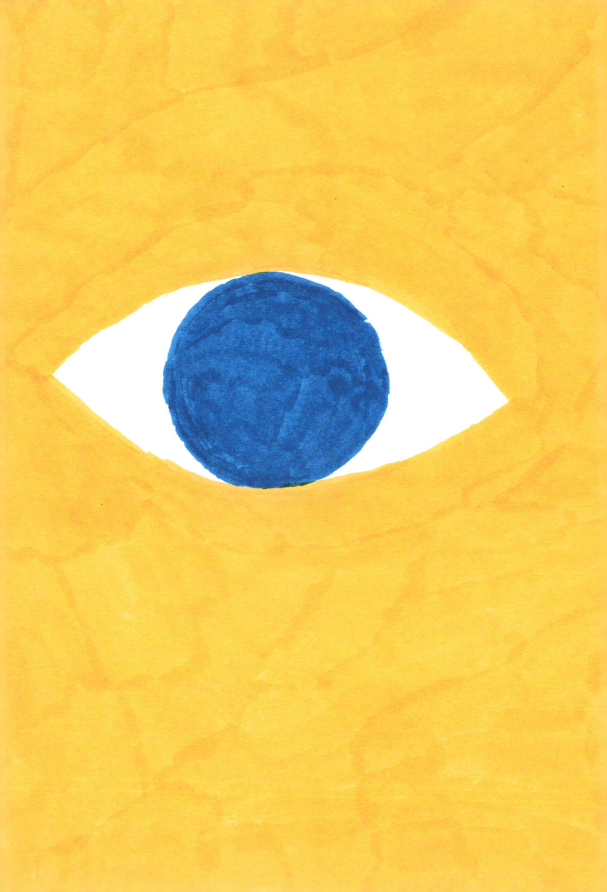

The Real Conversation Jesus Wants Us to Have

A Call to Bravery, Peace, and Love

Regina V. Cates

William B. Eerdmans Publishing Company

Grand Rapids, Michigan

Wm. B. Eerdmans Publishing Co.
2006 44th Street SE, Grand Rapids, MI 49508
www.eerdmans.com

© 2025 Regina V. Cates
All rights reserved
Published 2025

Book design by Lydia Hall

Printed in the United States of America

31 30 29 28 27 26 25   1 2 3 4 5 6 7

ISBN 978-0-8028-8410-7

Library of Congress Cataloging-in-Publication Data

A catalog record for this book is available from the Library of Congress.

Biblical quotations are from the New Revised Standard Version, updated edition, unless otherwise noted.

This book is dedicated to Lois Hanna Lawless and Jean and Reagan Cates, who love me as Jesus loves me.

I'm a little pencil in the hand of a writing God, who is sending a love letter to the world.
—Mother Teresa

Contents

	Foreword by Paula Stone Williams	ix
1.	Jesus Wants Us to Have This Conversation	1
2.	We're Never Supposed to Talk about This Topic	12
3.	We Need to Confront Beliefs That Cause Us to Be Uncomfortable	23
4.	Religious Dogma Is Ancient	32
5.	Religion and Morality Are Not the Same Thing	48
6.	They Are Us and We Are Them	59
7.	Sometimes We Turn the Other Cheek and Other Times We Don't	68
8.	Men of Quality Respect Women's Equality	78
9.	We Need to Talk about Sex	90
10.	Superheroes Are Real	108
11.	United We Stand	121

CONTENTS

12.	Racism, It's Time for Our Come-to-Jesus Moment	136
13.	We Are Part of God's Big Family	154
14.	To Heal, We Must Feel	166
15.	Love One Another as Jesus Loved	179
16.	Love Has Excellent Vision	189
17.	Care about the Legacy We Leave	200
	Acknowledgments	209
	Notes	211

Foreword

The book in your hands is dangerous if you want to stay stuck in one place. Regina Cates will make you question your beliefs and rethink your values as your faith grows and evolves.

As a pastoral counselor, people often come to me for help getting unstuck. My education is similar to that of other therapists, with an added spiritual dimension. For whatever reason, most of my clients do not come for spiritual counseling. They are looking for insight.

We humans are an inherently spiritual species, and if we do not address the spiritual dimension of our lives, insight will be elusive. Since most of my clients do not identify with any religion, I tiptoe into the waters of spirituality. I find most are stuck in the fourth stage described by James Fowler in his 1981 book, *Stages of Faith*.

Fowler's work is the spiritual equivalent of Piaget's theory of cognitive development, Eriksen's stages of psychosocial development, or Kohlberg's stages of moral development.

The first stage of faith is fluid and centered on parents and experiences. The second is literal, with a fixation on superheroes and justice. Fowler's third stage is conventional faith, adopting the religious ideals of one's family of origin, and seeing religion as rules and regulations. This is the realm of all religious fundamentalism and Christian evangelicalism. It is heavy on God's judgment and rooted in fear of eternal punishment.

Stage four is a time of angst, ennui, and struggle, as the individual grows beyond dualistic thinking. It often begins during one's college years, though if one is raised as an evangelical Christian, it can begin much later, if ever. I have a friend who calls this the stage of disenchantment. Because of the binary categories of evangelicalism, this can also be a period of rejection and exclusion. Those who remain in stage three are often fearful, and their commitment to their religious community can override their allegiance to family. When that happens, stage four can be very lonely.

Fowler's stage five is a time of reenchantment, in which the individual comes back to a vibrant spirituality, broader and deeper than before. The person is able to embrace paradox and mystery, and gain an appreciation of multiple faith traditions. Fowler calls stage six a universalizing faith, seeing all people as worthy of being treated with love and justice.

A few of my clients get stuck in stage three. Afraid of losing connections to friends and family, they acquiesce and put blinders on their expanding consciousness until it no longer is sustainable. For LGBTQ+ people, that moment arrives when they can no longer deny their inborn sexual or gender identity, and decide to live in concert with their core being. For others, their intellectual curiosity finally wins out over the need to belong. Or to put it in Jungian language, the Self triumphs over the ego. The ego is inordinately focused on safety and power. The Self is here for the ride, taking in the expansiveness of the human experience.

Stage four is always difficult. As I often say, the truth does set you free, but it makes you miserable first. If we are willing to accept

Foreword

the truth that the only way through the desert is to put our heads down and keep moving forward, our persistence is rewarded with the abiding peace and purpose that arrive with stages five and six.

While my clients raised in evangelicalism tend to get stuck in stage three, afraid of losing family, community, and salvation, my clients raised outside of religion get stuck in stage four. They not only have rejected religion; they have rejected their own spirituality, forcing its essence underground, where it is less likely to consider the Christian narrative and more likely to attach to less common spiritual expressions, like astrology, crystals, or Tarot cards.

We all need help moving from one stage to another. *The Real Conversation Jesus Wants Us to Have* is a great guide for those navigating the stages of faith, particularly those transitioning out of stage three and into stages four and five. Regina Cates invites us to examine the words of Jesus in context, as they relate both to Scripture and to our current cultural environment. Her own journey, painful, poignant, and redemptive, is a source of encouragement and a reminder that all who enter the desert can find an oasis and the courage to keep moving in the direction of wholeheartedness and hope.

To arrive at Fowler's stages five and six is to arrive at a place that looks like it has been expecting you. *The Real Conversation Jesus Wants Us to Have* will move you in the direction of that place, reminding you that you are not alone; others have been here before. And their guidance is incalculably helpful as we all seek to save the only life we can save.

Rev. Dr. Paula Stone Williams
Pastoral Counselor
Author of *As a Woman—What I Learned about Power, Sex,*
and the Patriarchy After I Transitioned

1

Jesus Wants Us to Have This Conversation

The longing to share my heart on the following pages was born in Rome, one of my favorite cities. Two friends and I once shared a memorable afternoon of candid and enlightening conversation in the Eternal City, surrounded by beautiful architecture, profound history, and delicious food. I credit it, these many years later, as the motivation for this book: part memoir, part social commentary, part call to action, and complete labor of love for Jesus.

After a morning visit with our tour group to view Michelangelo's fresco on the ceiling of the Sistine Chapel and his magnificent sculpture the *Pietà* housed in St. Peter's Basilica in Vatican City, my friends Barbara and Lisa and I decided to forgo a group trip to the Roman Forum in favor of spending some quiet time together. We strolled the vibrant city streets close to our hotel and eventually landed at the outdoor Caffe Portofino on the Piazza Cola di Rienzo. Over the next four hours we sipped coffee, treated ourselves to scrumptious pastries, and openly shared with one another.

We talked of heartbreak and joy. We spoke of goals achieved and those that remained elusive. We took on world events, politics, and religion. When late afternoon turned to early evening,

CHAPTER 1

we arrived at the topic of which famous person, living or dead, we would most like to engage in conversation.

Barbara is Jewish, yet she readily agreed with Lisa and me, who were raised Christian, it would be thrilling to have a discussion with Jesus. The *Pietà* inspired our unanimous choice. We could not imagine anyone not being deeply and permanently affected by the magnificent, lifelike sculpture of Mary cradling the dead body of Jesus. Mary is young. She is seated with Jesus laid out upon her lap, holding him with a loving, palpable anguish and a love so honest it moves one to tears simply by bearing witness to the enormity of her loss.

Michelangelo masterfully captured the lifeless body of Jesus in such a realistic way that every muscle and vein is visible. Such detail makes the death of Jesus by crucifixion real, troubling, and painful. I don't think any of us can imagine the depth of Jesus's emotional, psychological, and physical suffering—the beatings; the crown of thorns; being nailed to a cross to hang until dead; and the ridicule, denial, humiliation, betrayal, slander, and persecution he endured to bring a message of compassionate love to the world.

The *Pietà* is an exquisite expression of beauty and sorrow. To be in the presence of this loving tribute to Jesus and to Mary's sacrifice is to experience a deeply spiritual moment. It certainly motivated us to wonder what it would be like to sit with Jesus. What feelings would arise from being in his company? Gratitude, profound admiration, and affection, certainly.

What questions would we ask him? *During your last hours did you ever lose hope? Regret that you rocked the boat? Become angry? Doubt yourself? How did it feel to see your mother watching you die this way?*

While fantasizing about a conversation with Jesus, none of us considered Jesus might have many questions for us as well.

Jesus Wants Us to Have This Conversation

I believe the majority of us today, no matter our religious affiliation or lack thereof, would jump at the opportunity to sit down with Christ. I also think it is a safe bet many of us would not imagine an exchange with him to be anything but a love-filled, mostly one-sided talk of peace, forgiveness, and goodwill.

However, over the years since my trip to Rome—and having endured and witnessed religious, social, and political persecution and hypocrisy all my life—I have thought a great deal about what Jesus's side of a conversation with us would be like. Would Jesus's talk be love-filled, full of peace, forgiveness, and goodwill? Absolutely! I am also confident an engagement with the man who was a superhero of light in a dark world would be quite thought provoking and at times challenging. We must remember Jesus confronted the corrupt, power-hungry religious and political leaders of his day. He courageously opposed systematic persecution and rampant abuse of the marginalized of society by those in power. As a fair and honest person who was devoted to equity and social justice, he angrily overturned the tables of dishonest and greedy bankers in the temple who he believed did not belong there.

Jesus often exercised tough love, which means no matter how we may prefer to believe otherwise, he did get angry with those who lied, were dishonest, and abused others. Therefore, with all the turmoil, disinformation, and abuses of power in the world today, can we really think candid and honest Jesus would choose to stick with only polite and safe conversation?

I don't believe so.

Jesus was not afraid to initiate hard, tough-love conversations. He was not afraid to confront long-entrenched views. It was his confronting the misuses of power, illogical beliefs, and injustices he witnessed that ultimately led to his illegitimate trial and execution. By acknowledging his readiness to challenge behavior

CHAPTER 1

hurtful to his heart, we can be confident Jesus would not limit his conversation with us to only those topics of gracious engagement that everyone feels good about but is not necessarily improved by. We must remember: Jesus got into "good and necessary trouble," as civil rights giant and US Representative John Lewis put it.

Jesus, who was born around 6–4 BCE, died by crucifixion around 30 CE because he was seen as a threat to the Roman ruler, Tiberius, and to the authority of the governor of Judea, Pontius Pilate, and the religious leaders of his time. As the inspiration for Christianity, one of the world's major religions, he is also referred to as Christ, the Lamb of God, and the Prince of Peace. He remains the ultimate superhero to hundreds of millions of people throughout the world.

Why?

For many today, it is because Jesus knew how it felt to be an outcast from what was considered acceptable to those with religious, political, and social power. He resonates because he was persecuted in part for accepting those who were different.

Jesus was poor, which caused him to have deep compassion for the underprivileged and hungry. He struggled to make sense of social and religious structures that kept the moneyed and powerful in charge of everything and everyone. Today we continue to wrestle with a money-is-power-and-influence idea of success, intelligence, and entitlement.

Yet we are told it was the poor and humble shepherds who were among the first to acknowledge who Jesus was. They, the marginalized, outcast, uneducated, and needy of society, affirmed him. This affirmation from the disenfranchised provides us a glimpse of his entire mission on earth: to spread the message of valuing all of humanity. Not for beauty, riches, or power, but for what is truly wealthy about us to a loving God—kindness,

Jesus Wants Us to Have This Conversation

acceptance of the vast difference in all creation, and respect for all as equal.

Jesus resonates with some of us because, as he did, we too experience religious persecution.

He was a Jew who believed in one God—a belief that went against ancient Roman religion, in which people recognized and worshiped multiple gods and goddesses. He rejected not only multiple gods but also people playing at being God themselves. This caused him to courageously challenge those who abused their positions of religious power and twisted their beliefs to persecute others.

It was the abuses of power that caused Jesus to be an especially passionate champion for the marginalized of society. His life and teachings reflect the respect he had for all people's individual liberty and dignity. He demonstrated compassion and showed we can change the world for the better. He taught by example the spiritual and principled significance of living as people of honorable character, no matter the personal sacrifice involved. Rather than desiring wealth, fame, or power, he was devoted to being of loving service—something he demonstrated with humility when he washed the feet of his disciples.

Jesus's challenge to all who profess to love and follow him always was, and remains, that we strive to walk in his footsteps in daily life.

But are we actually building the respectful relationships and peaceful, cooperative, and sustainable world Jesus, the Prince of Peace, desired we create?

I don't believe we are.

However, I believe we can.

To do so, we must ask and answer thought-provoking questions about the inequity, injustices, and judgment we allow

CHAPTER 1

within our religious experiences, which help to increase, rather than decrease, divisive and abusive social interactions. We bravely speak truth to power. We set firm boundaries against abuse of all kinds. We distance ourselves from those who are driven by greed, spew disinformation, and are spiritually corrupted by their distorted view of Jesus.

We acknowledge that Jesus's challenge is for us to value, above everything else, the understanding that the joy, peace, and fulfillment we desire come from appreciating the vast world God created and from treating everyone and all life as we want to be treated.

He would challenge us to question why anyone who professes to love him would participate in or ignore behavior that is not aligned with his compassionate, respectful, and nonjudgmental heart. Jesus would want to know why many people who say they love him cause pain to others—often in the name of God.

After all, *Jesus specifically asked us to love our neighbor as ourselves.*

For me, this is the bottom line of what it means to be Christian—anyone (churchgoing or not) who strives to live Christ's example of compassion and integrity. Each day. In every way. With everyone.

The truth is, there is a vast difference in how Christians follow Jesus. Many do strive to walk in the loving-their-neighbors-as-themselves footsteps of Jesus. To give the hungry something to eat and the thirsty something to drink. To make friends of strangers. To care for the sick and visit those in prison. To clothe those in need. To love others as Jesus loves them. Christlike Christians live with the compassionate understanding that we are all one in the eyes of Jesus.

Many other dogmatic, Bible-thumping "Christians" love the Bible more than they love their neighbor. They defend judgmental beliefs rather than the oppressed. They have become comfortable abusing, in Christ's name, anyone they consider "other." I believe Jesus would want us to talk openly and honestly about the hypocrisy, domination, and confusion that are thriving within the religion founded in his name. Jesus would remind us that wounding others in his name is wounding him. To stop hurting Jesus, we must accept that we will never create the world he envisioned for us if we continue to deny or excuse the world in which we live.

As you turn the pages of this labor of love for Jesus, maybe my experiences and observations will resonate with you. Perhaps you will feel your experience is different. Possibly you will realize you have not evaluated your religious, political, and social involvement, or the experience of other people, from Jesus's perspective as a messenger of love, peace, and equity.

Regardless, shouldn't all who say we love Jesus be uncomfortable with the fact that fear, judgment, control, abuse of power, division, and self-loathing are being forced upon so many of us in his name?

I believe we must care enough to ask ourselves the questions I imagine Jesus may ask as part of this labor of love. I am confident he would absolutely care that people have always been, and are still being, persecuted and dominated in his name. I believe Jesus, who was a victim of the judgmental wounding and persecution of others, would not be okay with his name and memory being used to justify wounding and persecuting anyone.

We need to have the conversations Jesus wants us to have, because *Jesus did not turn the other cheek to abuses of power*. He stood up to those who oppressed others. He demonstrated that living with integrity creates our best life. He was positive and inclusive. He was trustworthy, honest, and nonviolent. He considered women his equals. He was empathetic. He acknowledged people by listening with his heart. He loved unconditionally. He assured everyone they were worthy of love.

Jesus's message to the world promoted the benefits of living with honesty, responsibility, and kindheartedness. So to truly honor Jesus, we need to confront the ways we, as Christians, too often abandon living Christ's example of compassion and honor. We need to examine whether we are giving our power away to those who are influential in religion, business, and politics who use Jesus and Christianity as weapons of control over us and others. The goal for each step we take is to think, behave, speak, and love as Christ did so he is proud to call us "friend."

If we don't equate being Christian with being Christlike, we must consider whether it is hypocritical and inaccurate to call ourselves *Christ*ians. The divine prince of peace, Jesus, reminds us that the wounded state of our outer world, both personal and collective, is a candid reflection of being disconnected from our kind, wise, peaceful, and loving heart.

These statements may feel confrontational. I get it. Facing the truth about our religious heritage is challenging. It is not easy to accept the discomfort we feel when confronting our limited beliefs, to expand our thinking about who we are and our reason for being, or to acknowledge that we are not loving one another as Jesus loved us.

We prefer to engage with pleasant, feel-good stories. It is easier to go down the path of disengagement and simply dismiss me, a messenger, as angry, misguided, wrong, a "lib," or a culture-war rebel rather than bravely consider the message. It is more comfortable to ignore what we don't want to face. We want to see ourselves as we believe we are, to comfort ourselves with thoughts such as "I'm not one of *those* Christians," or "We're doing God's will," or "The Bible is the final word of God," rather than look

Jesus Wants Us to Have This Conversation

at our religious indoctrination honestly, as if Christ were sitting next to us.

But to help create the world I believe Jesus envisioned for us—the one for which he made the ultimate sacrifice—we cannot retreat into the comfort of an existing mental framework like believing there is nothing we need to change about our attitudes and behavior or we don't need to question "our" beliefs: that sin is anything other than a negative choice we make over and over (like adultery, abuses of power, corruption, lying, etc.). That hurtful judgments about and domination of others are something *other* churches or religions do, not our own. That we must turn the other cheek and not speak out against abuse or challenge what other people believe, no matter how abusive those beliefs.

To truly love Jesus, we need to get into "good and necessary trouble." We need to get angry, as he did, with all that is not aligned with his love, to such a degree that we are moved to rise up and put an end to unloving, oppressive behavior that is considered acceptable in his name.

Jesus wants us to be brave, to face the often painful truth of our actions rather than comfort ourselves with lies. Let's be willing to be hurt by the truth. Let's remember, Jesus was hurt with lies. We are being hurt with lies, too, that are committed in his name. We must remember we are not to steal, or lie, or deceive one another (Leviticus 19:11 NIV). We owe him, and ourselves, thoughtful and honest deliberation as we face facts we are instructed to absolutely never talk about in polite society: facts about sex, abuse, religion, racism, white privilege and supremacy, bigotry, prejudice, gender inequality, politics, xenophobia, slavery, human sexuality, and our mental health. At the same time, religiously and politically motivated campaigns of fear and oppression seek to limit the

CHAPTER 1

rights of women to choose their own health-care options, to deny the human rights of members of the LGBTQIA+ community, and to keep entrenched within society systemic racism, white privilege, male dominance, and other forms of oppression. We must be willing to be hurt by the truth—Christianity should never be used as a weapon against anyone.

With so much fear, division, inequity, abuse of power, corruption, disinformation, and mayhem in the world, it seems Jesus's simple request to us, to love our neighbors as ourselves, is actually very hard to live by.

Why is that?

I have a theory.

Simply proclaiming oneself to be Christian and actually striving to love each other as Jesus loved us are enormously different approaches to following Jesus. Such different approaches exist because over two thousand years after his death, Western Christianity largely remains shackled to archaic, fear-based, and controlling religious dogma that does not, and never did, align with Christ's heart or his teachings.

I want you to understand this labor of love for Jesus was not easy for me to write. I know this "tough" love letter to fans of Christ may not always be easy to read. Some people may feel overwhelmed and angry. Some may simply want to reject these questions I propose Jesus would ask because these topics are often blunt, painful, and challenging.

No matter how uncomfortable or challenging it may be, *wouldn't our greatest act of love for Jesus be to examine Christianity, ourselves, politics, and society from his viewpoint?*

Let's imagine Jesus sitting across from us. It is just Christ, you, and me. Let's support one another in refusing to turn the other cheek to what is uncomfortable. Let's focus on what we

Jesus Wants Us to Have This Conversation

have to gain rather than what we might be challenged to give up. Let's demonstrate our love for Jesus by asking and answering the questions I imagine he would ask. And let's keep in mind that the following pages are offered out of a deep love for Jesus. I believe to truly follow him, it is imperative we help create the caring, peaceful, and respectful world he envisioned.

Doing so will require us to stop waiting for Jesus to show up and rescue us and to accept that he is waiting for us to rescue ourselves.

How?

By accepting such wisdom as that of author Brené Brown in her book *The Gifts of Imperfection*: "Only when we are brave enough to explore the darkness will we discover the infinite power of our light."[1]

God's loving grace within our heart is the power of light that gives us strength to honestly examine the oppressive attitudes and behaviors alive within much of Christianity—attitudes and behaviors that, to Jesus's heart, would not be either logical or kind. I believe Jesus would ask us to look at these attitudes and behaviors closely for the reason that just as a child's behavior reflects on their parents, the controlling and detrimental beliefs of some Christians reflect on all of Christianity.

I believe to help heal a wounded world, Jesus would want all Christians to be on the same page about what it means to follow him. He would tell us the universal mission of Christianity is to lead us, by example and teaching, to love our neighbors as ourselves. And he would challenge us to challenge ourselves to do so.

2

We're Never Supposed to Talk about This Topic

Spoiler alert: The topic we're never supposed to talk about is religion.
Why is that?
I have a pretty good idea.
I was brought up in a church that taught God is angry, vengeful, and male and I am an unworthy sinner going to hell for simply being born different—gay. There, with Satan, I will suffer eternity roasting on the devil's fiery spit.
Eternity is forever. Forever is hard to imagine.
To make it easier for children to visualize burning in hell endlessly, a Sunday school teacher told my class to imagine a turtle. It picks up one grain of sand in its beak on the Atlantic Ocean side of the United States, then slowly walks all the way across the country and puts the grain of sand down on the beach at the Pacific Ocean. The turtle then picks up a grain of sand from the West Coast and turns around to walk all the way back to the East Coast. One grain is deposited and another picked up. Over and over, the turtle schleps one grain of sand back and forth, for eternity.
I was terrified.

We're Never Supposed to Talk about This Topic

I have often thought of this and asked myself, Why is fear promoted in the very name of Jesus Christ: Christianity?

Could this help explain why we are warned to never, ever challenge our spoon-fed but often spiritually wounding religious beliefs or pastors, priests, ministers, and the Bible?

Isn't fear being intentionally used as a method of control?

When I was a young girl, attempting to accept such limited and disparaging ideas caused me so much anxiety, so many feelings of unworthiness, and so much shame that I lived in constant fear. It felt as if I were slowly being crushed beneath the oppressive weight of powerlessness and hopelessness. Of course I could avoid that hellish fate by being a good, straight girl; if I did, I would go to heaven instead.

Heaven would be a place of splendor where the streets are lined with gold. Peace and love would rain down. With God, I would spend a beautiful and much cooler eternity.

Around age seven, I found myself confronted with an enormous dilemma: I did not want to roast over hot coals, yet I had absolutely no hope of going to heaven, since it was certain I would never, ever gain acceptance there. God was in heaven, and God hated anyone who was gay, I had been clearly told. As young as I was, I knew I was different, and although I kept quiet about it, the gay-bashing messages from the pulpit and in Sunday school class left me with no doubt I was going to hell. I was taught being LGBTQIA+ is an intentional choice to sin against God. A choice? What child would intentionally put themselves in the crosshairs of religious and social hate? What adult would do so, for that matter? No one seduced me into being "gay." I just knew I was different but did not know why. When I began to ask questions, I was told a gay woman in church would have to have an operation to change from being gay. I did not want to have an operation,

CHAPTER 2

so hell it would be, as there was no winning a spot in heaven for me—which caused me to wonder, *How is a frightful, vengeful, judgmental God any different from Satan?*

To create a life of authenticity, self-respect, and love, I had to confront the fear, judgment, and contradictions I was exposed to in my religious experience that made no sense to my soul. I had to ask hard questions and challenge negative beliefs and practices out of life-saving necessity, since the entire fear-based, controlling, heaven-versus-hell, fall-in-line-or-be-damned indoctrination made no sense.

As you can imagine, as a child *without* power or voice, and *with* a big secret, I did not want to go to church. Yet I was made to go on Sunday morning and Sunday night with a midweek tune-up session on Wednesday and another on Friday night.

I had to read endless Bible verses about people who hated anyone who was gay . . . which meant they hated me. I was made to sing "Jesus loves the little children, all the children of the world." However, it was made clear Jesus did not love me.

With each verse of "Amazing Grace," my disgust for God, the church, and those who loathed me for simply being born different grew. Even if they didn't know yet that they hated me, I did. I was not blind. I clearly saw there was no saving a wretch like me.

Week after week, month after month, year after year, I was forced to sit in silence and expected to accept, without protest, all I was being taught. And I wondered, *Why aren't Jesus's love, inclusion of difference, and compassion the universal, Christlike message of Christianity?*

With no one to confide in, I lived in constant emotional isolation. I was sick all the time and depressed. I did not want friends. I preferred to be alone with my only true childhood companion, a doll named Doris. She and I retreated into our own world filled

We're Never Supposed to Talk about This Topic

with superheroes who saved people like me from injustice, pain, Satan, and a cruel God.

Doris became my playmate and confidant. She also served as a safe outlet to express the seething rage I had for life. I would hang Doris on the clothesline pole. I would stab her with a knife. I would punch her and drag her around the backyard by her neck.

I abused her. Yet I found no release in the mistreatment of the doll, since I cared for Doris, too. No matter how much I battered her, she offered a perpetual smile—I knew too well how that felt. In her gaze I found a protected space to share the depths of personal hell in which I already lived.

Knowing I was gay as a young child gave me a head start on a life of suffering. I cannot tell you how I knew so early on, but it is not uncommon for some gay, bisexual, and transgender people to know their orientation as young as five or six. Being gay was a secret I kept as long as possible. I knew exactly what would happen if I dared to tell anyone; I had been thoroughly schooled in how much "that kind"—my kind—was despised and feared. Feelings of unworthiness and shame steadily grew into blame, anger, and helplessness. I lived in constant fear of my secret getting out. I became a horrible student, unable to concentrate on anything other than the day I would begin my eternal confinement in Satan's inferno and the poor turtle would begin its never-ending, back-and-forth, sand-carrying journey.

In a desperate attempt to compensate for being gay and bad in the eyes of the church and society, I did everything possible to be worthy. I couldn't earn love through my grades, but I was frantic to win approval any other way I possibly could.

I got up early on Saturday mornings to clean the house. I mowed the lawn without being asked. I volunteered to take my grandmother shoe shopping. I excelled at sports and in band.

CHAPTER 2

I did what I was told. Yet no matter what I did or how polite I was, it was never, ever going to be enough. It made me think, *Why do we believe we can create heaven for ourselves while creating hell for others?*

Fear-filled dogma shamed me into living as a terrified, unworthy, and damned person.

As you can imagine, it was an absolutely horrible way to live.

Maybe you can relate. Maybe you are straight, or Black, or male, or disabled—maybe your experience in the world is different in any number of ways from mine—and yet you know exactly how I felt.

If you *don't* think my experience is the same as yours, I would encourage you to take a step back and honestly ask, *Would a kind, inclusive, and supportive Jesus truly feel at home and safe in your church? Would he be comfortable with the messages being delivered in his name?*

I am pretty sure the answer would make Jesus mad.

One day in my late teens, I got fed up with living in such terror and dread. I was told God would love me if only I were not gay—if only I were a good, straight, obedient girl. *Wait a minute,* I thought, *how can God love unconditionally and conditionally at the same time?*

It is either one or the other; it cannot be both.

The crazy-making, illogical, push-me-pull-me dogma of my Christian indoctrination was so overwhelming, I considered suicide. But instead of giving up on life, I chose to do the hard work of confronting why so much of what I was taught did not feel loving, logical, or right to my soul—or what I believe would be loving, logical, or right to Jesus. Fear and hostility are not in alignment with the God who loves unconditionally.

As Richard Rohr, a Franciscan priest and spirituality writer, observes, "We worshipped Jesus instead of following him on his

We're Never Supposed to Talk about This Topic

same path. We made Jesus into a mere religion instead of a journey toward union with God and everything else. This shift made us into a religion of 'belonging and believing' instead of a religion of transformation."[2]

Similarly, Reverend Benjamin Cremer, campus pastor at the Cathedral of the Rockies, wrote in a post on X: "I used to think taking Jesus' name was to say 'Jesus' as a cuss word. Now I think it is when we Christians demonize, condemn, and mistreat people in the name of Jesus all while ignoring his teaching in our own lives, our churches, our politics."[3]

My parents are Christian. As a child and young adult, I did not *choose* to adopt Christianity as my religion, just as I did not choose to be gay. Just as a child in India does not choose to be Hindu, or a child in Indonesia does not choose to be Muslim. Children around the world are innocent victims of generational religious indoctrination, meaning we are told what to believe, as our parents were and their parents before them. And like my parents and theirs, I was browbeaten into thinking if I challenged those beliefs, I was being blasphemous and going against God.

But what if the beliefs passed on to us intentionally dehumanize and abuse us or others?

Or cause us to live in fear rather than with Jesus's love?

If we want to stay in alignment with Jesus's heart, isn't it imperative to question our own hurtful beliefs and actions and those of others?

Emotional intelligence—the ability to put ourselves in the shoes of other people with empathy and respect—is the gift of God's grace to our soul. In order to benefit from this gift—to do no harm and to create a compassionate life—it is necessary to educate ourselves about the vast world God created versus our own limited thoughts and beliefs. We cannot rely on the groupthink that is generated by the thoughts and beliefs of an immediate

CHAPTER 2

circle of like-minded friends and family, one religious book, or a minister, infotainment celebrity, or political party. Wouldn't Jesus tell us not to give up thinking for ourselves—not to give our logic, problem-solving ability, and personal choice over to anyone?

If so, don't you imagine he might ask why there is so much fear about challenging beliefs or the controlling messages we hear within the religion created in Christ's name?

Asking ourselves to think deeply about the fact that "Christian" and "Christlike" are often two radically different things can be hard. Few of us can take an honest look at ourselves, our past actions, and our religious and political attitudes without feeling some degree of discomfort. Consequently, this means we tend simply to ignore those things about ourselves, our beliefs, and our world that are hard to face.

Yet refusing to tackle challenges head-on is leaving them to fester and grow more destructive and hurtful. The truth is, the messages we receive as children and from society to not talk about the "hard things" (such as religion, racism, and abuse) are control mechanisms designed to keep the status quo firmly in place. In order to heal our individual and collective wounding, we need to acknowledge and confront what it is we must heal.

If we just continue to sweep challenges under the rug, we will end up with a much larger lump that will eventually trip us, upending our entire lives and society.

We need to engage in honest conversation about what is going on within us and in our families, politics, and society. In order to move forward, we have to acknowledge the mistreatment we experience and witness, speak up against abuses of power as Jesus would, change for the better what is not aligned with his peaceful vision for us, truly honor his courage by being courageous ourselves, and answer these questions honestly:

We're Never Supposed to Talk about This Topic

Aren't the judgment and fear we encounter in our religious experiences increasing, rather than lessening, our divisive and abusive interactions?

Doesn't it make sense that when our religious experience is based on fear and unworthiness, we are intentionally being taught to live in fear and to feel unworthy?

Don't we need to admit that when we feel unworthy, we attempt to make ourselves feel worthy by scapegoating other people as the "unworthy" ones?

Let's ask Jesus to sit next to us in church, at home, and while we're on the internet or watching television. Let's ask him to walk with us through the hallways of government, the corridors of our schools, and the streets of our cities. I don't mean we scream his name or demand that others conform to our politicized version of him; I mean we need to bring his wise heart along humbly as we travel through life and engage with the world around us. The people in religious, political, and social authority who teach us our beliefs, dole out punishment and reward, and mirror society's behaviors may have labels like "pastor," "Supreme Court justice," or "influencer," but it does not mean we ought to blindly accept what they pass on to us as truth.

Jesus did not simply believe whatever those in positions of authority told him. He asked questions and challenged religious leaders and the practices of his time. Confronting the religious and political status quo is why Jesus was unjustly tried and executed. In his honor, and following his example, we have a moral obligation to heal the damage that was (and is still) being inflicted upon groups of people in Jesus's name.

One sunny afternoon, I was in my apartment working on this book when I noticed a man slowly walking up the steps of the neighboring building. His face was twisted in a scowl as he shuf-

CHAPTER 2

fled with head down, bent over under the enormous weight of an unseen burden. I watched him drop a pamphlet at each door. The little pieces of paper seemed immensely heavy in his hands.

An hour or so later, I went outside to find one of the booklets on my doormat as well. Across the front was written, "Are you saved? Where will you spend eternity?"

Without hesitation, I said out loud to no one, "With a little turtle."

I opened the pamphlet to find images of people burning in hell. There were threats that if I was not "biblically saved" (delivered by redemption from the power of sin and from the penalties ensuing from it) there was no hope of my ever getting out of hell. The fear-based, cruel, illogical religious beliefs of my hellish childhood are clearly still alive and being disseminated by many who represent Christ. *Wouldn't Jesus ask us to rise up and confront illogical ideas and nonloving treatment?*

Wouldn't Jesus want us to walk away from any religious, political, or social leader who desires to control our emotions through the use of anger, hate, or division? Through blame, lies, and fear?

I believe the answer is yes. I am confident Jesus would want us to confront everything we are exposed to that feels wrong to our loving and inclusive souls.

As spiritual beings on great human adventures, we are charged by our Creator with being ambassadors of God's loving grace, which means we help establish a positive and peaceful world for ourselves, our children, and their children's children. To accomplish our soul mission, the Divine gave us one simple and universal direction: Treat other people as you want to be treated.

Compassion—God's grace flowing through us—is the fundamental spiritual assignment for *all* world religions. To express God's grace as respect for one another, we must free ourselves

We're Never Supposed to Talk about This Topic

from the limitations of judgmental, punishing, and controlling religious dogma.

Let's accept that Jesus was a dark-complexioned Jew who practiced the Jewish tradition of *tikkun olam* ("repairing the world"). His mission on earth had nothing to do with having a whole new divisive religion created for him—and certainly not to have that religion misused in his name.

Therefore, let's wrap our hearts around the fact it was not Jesus's goal to install Christianity, as we know it in our modern, Western society, as the main religion of the world. It wasn't even Jesus's goal to establish the United States of America as his blessed and chosen nation.

We need to remember, or learn for the first time, a loving God gave the Golden Rule to all world religions and spiritual philosophies.

> Christianity; Matthew 7:12a: In everything do to others as you would have them do to you.
> Judaism; Elder Hillel in Babylonian Talmud, Shabbat 31a: What is hateful to you, do not to your fellow man.
> Islam; Abu Hamzah Anas bin Malik, Hadith 13, 40 Hadith an-Nawawi: Not one of you is a believer until he loves for his brother what he loves for himself.
> Hinduism; Mahabharata 5 (trans. Charles Wilkins): Do not unto others that which would cause you pain if done to you.
> Buddhism; the Buddha, Udana-Varga 5.18, Tibetan Dhammapada (trans. Sara Boin Webb): Whatever is disagreeable to yourself, do not do unto others.

This is not a complete list, as I have included only the world's five largest religions and spiritual philosophies. The ubiquity of

CHAPTER 2

the Golden Rule in so many faith systems throughout human history proves the same motivating Power was instrumental in the establishment of all of them.

Therefore, we must face the truth that there has been much confusion in Christianity about the desire to control the definition of God, the word of God, and the exclusive claim to what body of beliefs is most valuable to God. And the natural result of this confusion is an oppressive and illogical dogma about what one must do in order to be loved by God—or by us.

To love one another as Jesus asks, we must volunteer, out of love for Jesus, to perform deep spiritual investigation and searching for ourselves in order to establish a healthy balance between logic and love.

We cannot depend on other people to create our honest relationship with God for us. We cannot blindly accept what we are taught to believe in the name of God at the cost of condemning all others.

Simply agreeing without question is not an accountable or positive use of God's gift of free will. If something we hear sounds or feels off, we must listen to and act upon the ethical prompts of our souls.

Aren't these "twinges" of wisdom God's love speaking to us now, in real time?

Why do we think we can arrogantly dismiss the voice of logic and love inside our hearts when something does not feel right or we deem it unreasonable to our souls?

And this means we must have souls sensitive enough to detect dissent and brave enough to face discomfort.

3

We Need to Confront Beliefs That Cause Us to Be Uncomfortable

All Christians who look up to courageous Jesus must challenge their level of comfort with the uncomfortable that is promoted in Christ's name such as teaching that people with certain differences are going to hell. We must be willing to examine our comfort zones—which actually keep us *un*comfortable, and I have a theory about why.

We fear facing our fear.

Jesus taught love, not fear, but for too many of us, fear is a huge part of our religious experience, permeating our lives in both known and unknown ways until the uncomfortable becomes comfortable. We are so steeped in fear that it becomes normal—our baseline for existence. But let's remember, Jesus did not live in fear of anything—not failure, success, hell, death, strangers, or difference. He did not live in fear of being criticized, banished, or seen as a troublemaker. Jesus certainly did not fear causing trouble for those who caused trouble for others.

To honor him, we must not live in fear, either—which requires challenging ourselves to overcome our fear. Doing so demands self-love, self-respect, purposeful thought, and intentional effort.

CHAPTER 3

It also requires releasing the arrogant thinking that our beliefs are the only ones that are right, true, or divinely inspired, which often requires having our comfort zones shaken and having the safety of what is comfortable or familiar ripped away. To overcome our fears, we must confront our discomfort.

This happened for me on a hot summer day in middle Tennessee. Picture the scene: I crawl into the Lakota lodge on my hands and knees and find a place to sit. It is almost completely dark inside; the only light enters from a still-open doorway. There is just enough light to see I am with eleven people.

We form a circle on the dirt floor. We are so close to one another our knees touch.

No one speaks. The only sounds come from the hisses and pops of the fire burning outside.

Soon our leader enters and hangs an eagle talon over the door. He puts several objects close to him. One is a drum.

He breaks the silence by offering a prayer in English. When finished, he speaks to someone outside. A moment later, the first red-hot rock appears in the doorway. Using two sets of deer antlers, he picks it up and places the sizzling stone into a pit in the center of the room. Instantly the air grows hot.

When five large rocks, each about the size of my head, are safely inside the pit, thick blankets are pulled over the door. It is now completely dark inside. Our leader offers another prayer, then states the purpose of the Inipi ceremony. He assures us we can leave at any time, if we must. But he encourages us to stay, to face our fear and whatever discomfort comes up.

He asks us to form an intention for the ceremony: *What is it I want to gain from the experience?*

As I try to come up with an answer, he begins chanting in rhythm to a single drumbeat. I close my eyes. It is so hot. I am

We Need to Confront Beliefs That Cause Us to Be Uncomfortable

sweating. I try to pretend I am in a sauna, but even the first round of an Inipi feels hotter than a sauna.

After a few minutes, our leader's words and the drumbeat fade into the background of my consciousness. I feel myself begin to drift away. I open my eyes and cannot focus on my hand in front of my face. I cannot see anything other than a faint glow of the rocks and the wisps of steam that rise each time he pours water over them.

I shut my eyes tightly, trying to block out the heat. It does not work. I begin to wrestle with fear. I badly want to escape. I need to feel cool. Fear tells me if I don't get out now, I will never be cool again. I remind myself that isn't true, and that's when I begin to accept the truth: Fear tells us we may die if we face it head-on.

Fear creates endless reasons why I have to leave. And when I don't crawl out, fear digs deep. In the darkness of the Inipi lodge, surrounded by sweaty strangers and a Native American leader, my old religious dogma surfaces.

Hateful voices scream in my mind, *This isn't religious. It is sacrilege! It is pagan! It is the devil's work!*

I feel guilty, confused, afraid, and alone.

Then I hear someone crying. Fear briefly gives way to compassion. I cannot see who is crying, but I know we are both miserable and struggling.

The Inipi is designed to cause physical and emotional discomfort so that whatever comes up can be symbolically burned away. It works. While I am busy wrestling with fear and its urgent demands for me to get out of the lodge, bad memories begin to surface.

First, I see my sexual molestation by a babysitter and then a physician begin to surface. Then I am back in elementary school being bullied by a girl in a bathroom. I am sent to the principal's office and later punished by my parents. Even though I honestly

CHAPTER 3

stated my innocence, I am penalized for merely being in the wrong place at the wrong time. The memory reminds me I am wrong. I am always in the wrong.

Memories of betrayal, heartbreak, and pain come pouring into my mind. Inside the blazingly hot lodge, I return to abuse, persecution, and loneliness. And I wonder, *What if I can actually let go of resentment and blame?*

I cry. I appreciate the tears of my fellow lodgemates. Maybe some long-buried pain has surfaced for them, too. The onslaught of distressing memories is a complete shock to my system since I have not seriously thought of those experiences in years. When they had surfaced, it always seemed easier to ignore them, sweep them under the rug, refuse to face them head-on. *And what if by facing the fear of opening up hurtful wounds I can truly be free of past pain?*

Wading through upsetting memories, I am not aware how long we have been in the first round of the Inipi ceremony when the door opens. As intense light and cool air rush in, I feel drained, baffled, and a bit dizzy. I am sad and angry at being asked to confront my painful past. My eyes struggle to stay open against the brightness of the midsummer day. My head hurts from the heat; my heart hurts from the unexpected and unwanted emotional assault. It is hard to admit I had not forgiven or released the cruel treatment of my past.

I wipe my eyes. I feel self-conscious, like a child. For a brief moment I want my mother. I question my ability to withstand any more physical and emotional discomfort, but another part of me wants to continue since no counseling session, religious service, or confession to a friend has ever taken me so quickly down the path of confronting my fear and past abuse.

Do I have the courage to continue this spiritual awakening?

I decide to stay.

We Need to Confront Beliefs That Cause Us to Be Uncomfortable

The second round of rocks enters. The door closes, and the air becomes hotter than before. I focus on being more connected to the ceremony this time around.

I join the other people in prayer. I sing. I voice my intent to be free of fear. I ask God to release my anger and resentment and rid me of the emotional pain of my past. I cry more. I remember more hurt and disappointment. I feel deep compassion for who I was in the past and what I endured. I sweat intensely. There is no piece of my clothing that is not soaking wet.

Another half hour passes.

When the door opens this time, I feel a bit lighter, a bit freer. I cannot explain how, but the physical and emotional suffering I am experiencing in the Inipi is replacing my fear and feelings of being victimized with courage, willpower, and strength. And I begin to understand: If we dare to confront the darkness we all carry, fear *can* fall away for good.

During the break I sit in silence and pray for forgiveness for those who wronged me. I also ask for forgiveness for all the wrongs I committed against others. It is important to me that I own my role in causing harm to others, too.

I pray to be free of self-importance. I ask to leave my self-centered ego—my wounded and unhealthy sense of self—inside the lodge. I ask to be filled with compassion and respect.

I ask God for guidance. I ask God to let me know beyond a doubt the difference between divine direction and self-righteous thinking.

I don't know how long the next round will be, and once again, fear briefly questions whether I can withstand any more. But I stay, determined to see this through.

More hot rocks are added to the center of the lodge as the third round begins. Stifling steam mixed with sage burns my

CHAPTER 3

lungs. It is uncomfortable, but I breathe deeply, focusing on the rhythm of the drum.

I am hotter than I have ever been in my life. I pray more. I release more emotion. More painful memories pass through my consciousness. I drink water from a passed cup. I sweat. I feel something profound happening within me, as if I am being purified. This Inipi is cleansing away years of fear, regret, and anger.

Another half hour passes.

The door opens a third time. Our leader says we can leave; we don't have to stay for the final round. There will be no shame or judgment.

A few people crawl out into the sunlight. I remain rooted in place. As the door closes for the fourth and final round, the Inipi begins to feel reassuring, as though I have come home after a lifetime of wandering, searching for a way to finally establish a loving and strong connection to God. It happens in a place I would not have dreamed possible—something so outside my history. And I learn the truth: being spoon-fed religion deadens our spiritual growth.

That experience in a Lakota sweat lodge would never have been permitted by the religion of my youth, even though it led me closer to the heart of God than years of sitting in a hard-backed pew with a hymnal in my hands. It took moving way beyond my comfort zone for me to recognize I could find God in other ways and, in so doing, cultivate a deep commitment to the continuous self-assessment necessary to maintain a personal relationship with Jesus. I had heard enough sermons to know how easy it is to passively receive from someone else—someone who claims to speak on behalf of God. It is much more difficult to do the day-to-day, moment-by-moment inner work of actively determining whether we are actually walking in the footsteps of Jesus's empathy and integrity.

We Need to Confront Beliefs That Cause Us to Be Uncomfortable

Most of us don't purposely seek out discomfort—it took an enormous amount of inner strength and courage for me to remain in the lodge that day—but when we allow ourselves to experience discomfort rather than hide from it, we can learn much more about ourselves than we ever imagined. It turns out, God really *does* help those who help themselves.

God's grace for us is constant and nonjudgmental, no matter how far we stray from the integrity and goodness of our souls. But God's grace does not release us from the responsibility to strive to live as the best version of ourselves. God's grace asks us to honestly face the consequences of choosing not to do our best. God's grace comforts and encourages us when we realize our mistakes can be lessons to do better next time. God's grace is patient in our learning process. The grace of God gives us the courage to step outside our comfort zone to ask hard questions because what is most important to God is the depth of determination we have to know ourselves as the souls we are—as eternal parts of our loving Creator—and how we will use that power to demonstrate the love of God to the world.

God helped me tremendously because I helped myself that day. Because I confronted fear and exchanged it for courage, I left the lodge with a new respect for the strength of my physical body—a body I had previously been taught was shameful and sin-riddled. Because I was willing to work through the complex emotions of past traumas, I made huge strides in gaining real emotional freedom from the buried pain that was still causing me to be less than my potential. I came away with a deeper reverence for all life, for myself, for God.

My concept of God began to move from a suggestion imposed on me by other people to a living experience of personal resonance. My willingness to ask hard questions and face my fears inspired

CHAPTER 3

a deep devotion to Jesus because of his compassion and love in standing by me. More than any prayer mumbled in a church or baptism in front of a congregation, this is what invited him to take up permanent and welcomed residence in my heart. By surrendering to the unknown of the Inipi ceremony, I learned that my comfort zone had actually been keeping me uncomfortable.

No Sunday-school class, hellfire-and-damnation sermon, or vacation Bible school ever enabled me to comprehend God as I began to that day. Not one religious experience I had came close to the profound spiritual awakening I began achieving inside a Native American sweat lodge. And I learned *we don't have to carry the title "Christian" to live a Christlike life.*

It is humbling to comprehend that what we call God was around long before human beings were human beings. God was around long before human beings created religions, labels, and beliefs about God and one another.

Retired American bishop of the Episcopal Church and bestselling author John Shelby Spong explained it this way: "God is not a Christian, God is not a Jew, or a Muslim, or a Hindu, or a Buddhist. All of those are human systems which human beings have created to try to help us walk into the mystery of God. I honor my tradition, I walk through my tradition, but I don't think my tradition defines God, I think it only points me to God."[4]

How can we know what God is?

We are told what God is, but the truth is, we cannot put infinite God into a form or gender.

To me, God smells like a rainy day. God feels soft, like the fur of a kitten. God sounds like songbirds. God looks like spring, summer, winter, and fall. God is every act of forgiveness, compassion, and respect. I believe the best way to view God is to see God intentionally in everything and everyone, because that motivates us to treat all people and all life as we want to be treated.

We Need to Confront Beliefs That Cause Us to Be Uncomfortable

But just as an advanced degree requires years of study in a variety of disciplines and subjects (even if we ultimately specialize in just one), an expanded wisdom regarding God's divine design of the interconnectedness of all life is not the result of being spoon-fed a single viewpoint of truth. In all things, as our understanding and maturity grow, the reward is a wider breadth and depth of knowledge. Our skill levels increase, as do our deductive reasoning and critical-thinking abilities. Our values and priorities change. We develop our inquisitive natures. The more we question ourselves, our assumptions, and our traditions, the more we learn, grow, and change for the better.

By embarking on a journey of honest reflection, we can stand up and stand out as living examples of what Jesus would do because we have explored the nature of Jesus from many different angles. We understand more fully the motivations and impulses at the heart of his life and his example, and we are better prepared to accept the enormity of what it means to live as he did.

We love God, and we love as God asks us to, by being people of compassion and integrity because only when we remain aligned with the integrity and compassion of our souls are we aligned with God. In order to truly honor Jesus, we must challenge ourselves to overcome fear and live in love as he did. *Judgment Day is not some time in the future; it is now, today, this moment.* We are called *every single day* to live as Jesus asked us to—to measure our conduct against the standard he set for us in unambiguous terms. The question is whether we are willing to let go of our own personal comfort in order to do so.

4

Religious Dogma Is Ancient

The Bible was written thousands of years ago, yet too often what seemed true for societies back then is taken as absolute for our society today. Without considering the cultural context of the ancient societies that produced religious texts, we often take what is written literally. And when we consider ancient religious texts infallible and beyond debate, we are not willing to discuss our beliefs rationally.

This belief in the Bible's infallibility is the reason many Christians avidly fight against the human rights of so many people they consider to be "other" and "sinners," such as immigrants, people from other religious backgrounds, or the LGBTQIA+ community.

Many Christians find it hard to reconsider or let go of these beliefs, even when those beliefs conflict with new scientific knowledge or test a parent's love for their child. Like me.

At age eighteen I could no longer deny who I was, so I told my parents I was gay. With the intention of "curing" me, they sent me to a physician, who sexually molested me. Then I was locked in a psychiatric hospital because the physician and my parents thought I was depressed. *Of course* I was depressed. I had just been sexually violated, and the two people who were supposed to love me unconditionally told me I was going to hell and had broken their hearts.

Sadly, my parents' Christian religious experience taught them to detest gay people, while at the same time they had to make sense of contradictory messages, such as "Do not judge, so that you may not be judged" and "In everything do to others as you would have them do to you; for this is the law and the prophets." So when I confessed my big secret, they faced their worst nightmare: Which contradictory yet supposedly inerrant message should they embrace?

I am certain they believed their motivation was love. I'm sure they believed changing me to heterosexual would save my soul from eternal hellfire and damnation.

I am also certain my parents desired to escape being ridiculed and shunned themselves if my secret got out. They literally told me, "You're a business risk" and "Go live at the YWCA."

But Jesus-like love supports and comforts, so wouldn't a compassionate Jesus ask, "If we don't listen to the stories of the outcasts, or care about how our beliefs made them outcasts in the first place, isn't this living in a consequence-free ivory tower of self-righteousness?"

As a child, I fantasized about writing a letter to Christian pastors. I wanted to ask, among many other things, why they insisted their God hated me for being gay.

Many decades later, I was moved to initiate the conversation I had imagined. I wrote to thirty-one prominent Christian ministers from various denominations throughout the United States. I also sent my letter to His Holiness the Pope.

Only a handful responded. A few were polite; a few were not.

I received a respectful letter from the pope's representative, which I saved. I was also gifted with a set of audio tapes from a

CHAPTER 4

popular southern television evangelist telling me I was a sinner who was going to hell unless, of course, I changed my "choice" to be gay. Those I quickly trashed.

I also began a discussion with one West Coast minister, but our communication hit a wall when my response to what he had called our "welcomed conversation" was met with complete silence. When I countered his literal interpretation of the Bible, he apparently felt there was no reason to continue the discussion. He had warned me nothing would change his mind, but I was not even given the opportunity for our conversation to change his heart—the only part of us capable of loving one another as Jesus asks us to.

I will never forget the look of disappointment on my parents' faces when, after I had spent ten horrible days in the psychiatric hospital, a psychiatrist told them at a follow-up appointment he could not change my sexuality. "Like so many aspects of our uniqueness," he said, "human sexuality is not a choice one makes." There would be no praying or converting the gay away.

Hallelujah! For the first time ever, I felt acceptance and compassion. And it came from a complete stranger.

Was he Christian?

Who knows, but his support allowed me to gain a small sense of self-approval. I began to imagine I might be worthy of love after all.

However, the inner turmoil did not permanently resolve as a result of this one confirmation. I had no clue how to navigate the straight world as a gay member of our human family. I did not know how to love Jesus when my Christian religious experience told me God hates gays. I could not understand why my parents, or anyone who professed to love an accepting Jesus, could shun me simply for being different.

For many years I was estranged from my family. I was emotionally devastated by the holier-than-thou reasoning of those

Religious Dogma Is Ancient

who defended their condemnation of my sexual orientation, when Jesus himself did not say anything on the subject. Why were none of the adults in my life confronting the rampant contradictions in the version of Jesus they taught?

Waging war against others is not aligned with Jesus's message. Nor would he excuse my waging war against people who judged me. We were both operating contrary to what he taught. As a result, I suffered under the heavy burden of resentment and confusion as I struggled to reconcile my perceived sin (my sexuality) with my actual sin (my anger toward those who had harmed me)—a weight so massive it almost made me give up on life. I struggled with the painful reality that *all* judgmental, hurtful, and divisive messages delivered in God's name must be challenged.

The thing is, I know my parents always cared for me. They simply had no clue how to accept me while also following their religious convictions. Their religious experience (and mine, by extension) did not support challenging was what supposedly delivered in God's name. Maybe yours didn't, either. So let's honestly ask ourselves: *Why are we so fearful of challenging our pastors, investigating the origins of the Bible, or holding up what we are taught about God, Jesus, and the world against science?*

We have a tendency to view ourselves, other people, and the world around us through the lens of what we already believe to be true. However, when our goal is to live with an inclusive and loving heart, as Jesus desires us to do, we have a duty to challenge whether our limited beliefs accurately reflect the vast world God created. If we're fearful of honestly questioning and challenging our beliefs, doesn't that indicate a huge deficit of faith? Wouldn't Jesus ask us to humbly admit we don't know what we don't know and to open ourselves to expanding our perspectives rather than

CHAPTER 4

lying to ourselves or others simply because we don't want to admit we may not have all the answers?

The fifth-century Greek philosopher Socrates also encouraged people to focus on becoming aware of and responsible for our ignorance. He believed the beginning of wisdom was an awareness of one's own ignorance. When we admit our ignorance about ourselves, other people, history, science, and other topics, we open ourselves up to expanding our understanding rather than proceeding through life with a closed mind.

It is vital that we remember that being told something is true is not the same as it actually being true; likewise, being taught to believe something does not make that belief valid.

Yet we want our beliefs to be true. That is why, when our beliefs are challenged, there is a tendency simply to reject the messenger rather than bravely entertain the message and consider whether there is anything to it. However, by not confronting tough issues, we are denying our part in them. As long as we blame those we view as complainers and refuse to listen to their experiences and observations rather than allowing them to be heard and examined, we will maintain a status quo (our beliefs about God, ourselves, and other people) that often conflicts with the heart of Jesus.

I asked Tim Moody, my friend and a former Christian minister, why many Christians are fearful of asking hard questions of themselves and others. This is how he responded in an email I received in the fall of 2018:

> In most Christian churches, the minister is a fixed authority figure, above reproach. So they see little need or desire to question him (or, rarely, her). There is also the fact that many Christians see the Bible as completely sacrosanct, without

Religious Dogma Is Ancient

distortion, misrepresentation, or error of any kind. Consequently, some of the strong demands of the Bible, especially in the Old Testament, and in much of Paul's writings, are taken literally and without any hesitation. Without reasoning about context, background, geography, language, culture, and other vital components, which help us fully understand Scripture, believers have, over the years, developed notions about God and Christianity that don't reflect the biblical and historical account of who Jesus was and what he taught.

Everything is just accepted as true. And whole doctrines, rules of conduct, righteous actions, and Christian standards are created out of primitive ideas frozen in history. It is no wonder many Christians have never wrestled with the tough and complex issues of how the Bible was put together. Who actually wrote it, when was it written, and what do the indisputable contradictions mean?

Without addressing these complex issues, we fail to understand our own humanity, the power of free will, that we are never controlled by Jesus or the Holy Spirit or any other force except the consequences of our own choices.

The old rigid myths, the sanctimonious judgments, and the horrid distortions of who Jesus was and is are all a part of the misuse of Scripture. I witness how this misuse harms the Christian community as a whole and corrupts the actual love Jesus demonstrated for all people. I feel Jesus would view this judgmental approach to faith a clear misuse of Christianity's core mission and truth.

For us to treat people as we want to be treated, to reflect a loving God's grace, we must be willing to allow the thoughts and beliefs we have about the Bible and Christianity to be challenged.

CHAPTER 4

That doesn't even mean they need to be changed with every encounter; certainly there will be some who challenge more open beliefs with close-minded ones. But without a *genuine* (not performative) willingness to hear and consider these viewpoints, we will never learn, grow, and mature in our faith.

To be right with Jesus, we must be superheroes for him (as I imagined myself as a child creating a better world in the name of Christ) and focus our spiritual practice on demonstrating his inclusive love for the vast world the power we call God created. And that requires us to bravely scrutinize everything in our religious experience that is not aligned with Jesus's empathy, including ancient beliefs that are still being used to judge, dominate, and abuse people in Jesus's name. We need to focus on what we will gain by changing outmoded and incorrect beliefs rather than fear what we have to give up. We must appreciate that the Bible is bound by the societies and customs that prevailed when it was written.

We have a duty to educate ourselves to ancient practices that were the basis for Bible verses still being used today to shape and defend Christians' judgmental view of homosexuality and more. I am gay, and that is okay with God—even though there are seven "clobber" verses in the Bible about same-sex relations. We need to remember, biblical times were different from our own time.

There is a tremendous amount of scholarship on this topic for those who are willing to consider it. A devout Christian friend of mine discovered during research for her master's thesis in seminary that when nations waged war against each other in ancient times, the (male) soldiers often raped the losing army. This act of violence and humiliation toward the weaker nation seems to have been one foundation for the verses in the Bible about same-sex relationships.

Religious Dogma Is Ancient

Matthew Vines, an openly gay evangelical Christian and the author of *God and the Gay Christian: The Biblical Case in Support of Same-Sex Relationships*, provides other plausible historical explanations for verses in the Bible about same-sex relationships.[5] He writes:

> Paul uses two Greek words—*malakoi* and *arsenokoitai*—that likely refer to some forms of male same-sex behavior, but not the modern concept of homosexuality. The predominant forms of same-sex behavior in the ancient world were sex between masters and slaves, sex between adult men and adolescent boys, and prostitution. In all those cases, men used sex to express power, dominance and lustfulness, not self-giving love and mutuality. Committed same-sex unions between social equals represent very different values than the types of same-sex behavior Paul would have had in view in 1 Corinthians 6.[6]

None of the ancient Bible verses refer to LGBTQIA+ orientations as they are now understood. As modern biblical scholars advise us, the verses regarding same-sex relationships throughout ancient religious texts need to be kept within the context of the ancient societies that produced them. We understand the science of biology and genetics more fully now, and the medical, psychological, and educational communities of today acknowledge the impact of their role in sexuality.

Steven Novella, MD, executive editor of *Science-Based Medicine* and clinical neurologist and associate professor at the Yale University School of Medicine, writes, "Those who opposed gay rights in the past claimed (and some still claim) that homosexuality is a choice, or a product of social influences, perhaps even a mental disorder or pathology. Years of research have led to the conclusion that sexual orientation among humans is simply more fluid than old-school strictly binary concepts. People are heterosexual, homosexual, bisexual, pansexual (romantic feelings that are blind to sex or gender), asexual, and everything in between."[7]

Dick F. Swaab, MD, a professor of neurobiology at the University of Amsterdam, agrees: "Current evidence indicates that sexual differentiation of the human brain occurs during fetal and neonatal development and programs our gender identity—our feeling of being male or female and our sexual orientation as hetero-, homo-, or bisexual."[8]

Elliot Kukla, a rabbi, author, artist, and activist who is transgender and nonbinary, challenges those who use religion to push legislative agendas that limit the rights of LGBTQIA+ people:

> This legislative attack is often framed as a battle between traditional religious values and modern ideas about gender. But we [LGBTQIA+] are real people, not ideas, and we have always existed, including within age-old religions. In my own tradition, Judaism, our most sacred texts reflect a multiplicity of gender. This part of Judaism has mostly been obscured by the modern binary world until very recently.
>
> There are four genders beyond male or female that appear in ancient Jewish holy texts hundreds of times. They are considered during discussions about childbirth, marriage, inheritance, holidays, ritual leadership and much more. We were always hiding in plain sight, but recently the research of Jewish studies scholars like Max Strassfeld has demonstrated how nonbinary gender is central to understanding Jewish law and literature as a whole.

Religious Dogma Is Ancient

When a child was born in the ancient Jewish world it could be designated as a boy, a girl, a "tumtum" (who is neither clearly male nor female), or an "androgynos" (who has both male and female characteristics) based on physical features. There are two more gender designations that form later in life. The "aylonit" is considered female at birth, but develops in an atypical direction. The "saris" is designated male at birth, but later becomes a eunuch. There is not an exact equivalence between these ancient categories and modern gender identities. Some of these designations are based on biology, some on a person's role in society. But they show us that people who are more than binary have always been recognized by my religion. We are not a fad.[9]

Despite scientific and cultural evidence that gender-as-a-binary is *not* "the way it's always been," many people within Christianity and society in general are still taught that being lesbian, gay, bisexual, transgender, questioning, queer, intersex, pansexual, two-spirit (2S), androgynous, and asexual are choices, or that sexual identity is learned.

If this is true, the next logical questions are *When? How?*

If someone is raised in a system that threatens them with eternal damnation for being gay, why would someone intentionally choose to live under that crushing burden of an eternity in hell or even the temporary hell of endless bullying by society in general?

I never made such a choice. And yet, here I am—perfectly gay. *I was born this way.* And I am okay.

We are all born the way we are because of our genetic makeup. Certainly, there are other influences, such as our physical and social environment, that can influence the way we develop, but everyone exhibits traits based on their unique biological profile.

CHAPTER 4

Jesus said nothing about race or gender being important to save one's soul; in fact, he actively welcomed Samaritans, who were ethnically different from the Jews. Likewise, *Jesus never said heterosexuality was essential for salvation, either*. Saying sexual orientation or gender identity is a choice makes no more sense than saying racial or ethnic identity is a choice.

With logic and love, let's honestly consider this question: If a heterosexual orientation, and none other, is a central component to spiritual salvation, wouldn't God have said something along the lines of the following?

> Jesus, I'm going to need you to address the gay thing head-on. While you're at it, Son, go ahead and address transgender, bisexual, asexual, pansexual, lesbian, intersex, two-spirit, and a host of other biological circumstances, as these will come up in a few thousand years or so. And while you're on a roll, make clear my views on environmental destruction, the exploitation of workers, child labor, war as a business, the manufacturing and selling of weapons of war to civilians, the intentional mass incarceration of people of color, the fallacy of race, suppression of women, vilification of the press, misogyny, dictators, corruption, and the blatant disregard for the ever-changing landscape of scientific and intellectual knowledge. Got it? Good. We've already lined up a sermon on the mount and a sermon on the plain; maybe let's make this the sermon on the plateau.

Many Christians have moved beyond a creation of six literal days as well as the idea that any physical or emotional ailment is demonic in origin. Shouldn't the same apply for issues related to human sexuality?

Religious Dogma Is Ancient

I recognize it can be easier to reject scientific findings than to challenge the Bible and what we are taught to believe. Certainly there are mountains of evidence proving companies, governments, politicians, and individuals often readily reject scientific data when it threatens to negatively affect their beliefs or bottom line. Actions like these reflect the intentional, dishonorable choice to refuse ever-evolving information, to remain willfully ignorant, or to protect financial investments rather than care about their detrimental impact on people and the planet. Willful ignorance about human sexuality appears when religious communities and individual believers reject scientific evidence in favor of beliefs based on their interpretations of the Bible.

What many Christians don't realize, or don't want to admit, is that most of the Bible was written down from countless ancient oral traditions by men whose cultures—their language, practices, and knowledge base—were far removed from our own. What we have preserved in the Bible is the result of stories, traditions, and recollections that scribes recorded over centuries. Similarly, the New Testament of the Christian Bible was written two thousand years ago, in the first century CE. In the intervening millennia, countless interpretations of Scripture have emerged—and will continue to emerge—for as long as human beings engage with the text.

As John Dominic Crossan, New Testament scholar and former Catholic priest, observes, "My point is not that those ancient people told literal stories and we are now smart enough to take them symbolically, but that they told them symbolically and we are now dumb enough to take them literally."[10]

We must understand we can be good people and also be complicit in an unjust, illogical, and harmful system. We must accept that the key to changing any damaging system is to grow our empathy for the plight of other people. One way we do so is to accept that *Jesus did not write the Bible and was not alive when it was written.* Accepting that Jesus did not write the Bible allows us to bravely call out and separate ourselves from those who use their misguided beliefs to abuse anyone in the name of Christ.

Rather than blindly accepting the Bible without question, perhaps we should be engaging with the text in thoughtful and intellectually curious ways, asking questions such as, Why does it seem there was intentional editing of what we now know to be Scripture, to craft a specific message reported by those in religious power to be the infallible word of God or to portray Jesus in a certain way? Or if we are supposed to model our lives on the Bible, why is it often confusing and contradictory?

Since at least the nineteenth century, biblical scholars have recognized that each of the Gospels seems to have been composed with a different agenda and for a slightly different audience: Matthew for a Jewish audience awaiting the messiah; Mark to make the case for Jesus as the Son of God and the centrality of the crucifixion and resurrection; Luke as a historical account for gentile readers steeped in Greek culture; and John from the point of view of one of Jesus's closest disciples and with a broader worldview.

While the purpose of the Four Gospels may have been to record the life of Jesus, each author tailored his message for a certain group. The Gospels have similarities, but there are also contradictions, resulting in each Gospel having its own political and religious agenda. The books of Matthew and Luke, for example, present different accounts of Jesus's birth, while all four Gospels contradict each other about the resurrection.[11] It is also important to remember oral tradition formed the substance of the Gospels, the earliest of which was Mark, written around 70 CE, about forty years after the death of Jesus; in other words, these were not eyewitness, contemporary accounts composed in real time as Jesus was teaching. Additionally, all four books were published anonymously, but historians believe the books were given the name of Jesus's disciples or other early followers of Jesus to lend them greater authority.

Knowing this, shouldn't we keep in mind (when considering the Bible as the unchangeable and definitive word of God) that the Bible was written over a long period of time by different men who created messages based on their own personal vantage points? Is it not then responsible for us to recognize that over the intervening centuries, the "meaning" and interpretation of that same text could have continued to be crafted by those in positions of religious and political influence?

These are important questions to ask because, as Reverends Emily Swan and Ken Wilson remind us, "those most likely to be literate and viewed as theologically sound in the last five centuries have been white, male, educated and Western. This means that the translation and interpretation of Scripture has largely been handled by the category of people with the most power in the world over the last 500 years."[12]

Jesus, the enlightened soul and Jew, brought a modern message to a world whose only modes of transportation were by foot, boat, cart, or on an animal's back. Moonlight or oil lamps alone cast a tiny glow in darkened homes at night. Locusts were considered a delicacy.

The world has transformed in countless ways since Jesus's era. Yesterday's knowledge, understanding, and technology yield to today's. I don't believe Jesus would want us to ignore science about human sexuality, vaccines, the environment, scholarly research into the origins of and contradictions found within ancient religious texts, and so much more.

CHAPTER 4

Modern science and research matter to expanding our understanding of everything. We can't simply deny science and scholarship when they conflict with a religious belief. It is these conflicts that give us the opportunity to learn and grow.

By denying the findings of climate scientists or epidemiologists, aren't we refusing to engage as responsible stewards of the earth and the life it contains?

By not being responsible stewards of our environment, aren't we irresponsibly dumping our waste and toxic practices onto our children and theirs?

By denying scientific research about human sexuality, aren't we hurting ourselves, our children, and other people?

How can we justify dismissing scientists, religious scholars, historians, and archaeologists simply because their findings are uncomfortable or inconvenient to us? How do we engage in honest, peaceful, and respectful conversation with more traditionally minded Christians about how many of their judgments are based on antiquated beliefs and are in conflict with our modern knowledge of the nature of ever-expanding design—especially when entertaining such ideas is often regarded as politically motivated or morally dangerous?

Meteorologist and evangelical Christian Paul Douglas writes, "Being open to data, facts and science doesn't make you a liberal. It makes you literate. Scientifically literate. It means you favor data, facts, and evidence over conspiracy theories, manufactured information, and cherry-picked industry spins."[13]

What person (of any faith) is not appreciative of being connected to the Internet? Or does not rejoice when the mammogram results are clear, or when a blood test confirms the life-threatening illness has been eradicated?

Would Jesus, as a messenger of enlightenment, view our actions as loving if we embrace science that benefits us while

Religious Dogma Is Ancient

rejecting science that challenges our comfortable religious assumptions? To deny scientific indications that human sexuality has a biological component, yet to accept science that personally benefits us or a loved one (such as antibiotics, chemotherapy, or even just handwashing to reduce infection), is hypocritical, illogical, and self-serving thinking.

Was Jesus hypocritical, illogical, or self-serving?

Educated, we are less likely to be politically, religiously, or socially manipulated through misinformation. Education allows us to think critically and independently. I believe Jesus would appreciate that education is a lifelong process, and everything is designed to change and progress—the seasons, nature, scientific understanding, technological and cosmological discoveries, even human intellect.

All things are designed to change and grow, including our spiritual beliefs and practices. We have the duty to allow—even to encourage—our hearts and souls to evolve. Only by asking questions of ourselves and being open to advancement and transformation do we improve intellectually and technologically from generation to generation. Growing our spiritual understanding works the same way.

Spiritual advancement ensures we bring accountability, forethought, and principled excellence to the table when addressing challenges and opportunities—exactly as Christ has called us to do.

5

Religion and Morality Are Not the Same Thing

I am not comfortable calling myself Christian. As you can tell by now, I am a big fan of how Jesus lived and how I believe he asks us to live in order to create our best life, but I'm not a fan of the label.

Rather than tagging myself with the name "Christian," I go through life imagining Jesus beside me. My goal in every interaction is to make Jesus genuinely proud to call me a friend.

My friend Jesus was a man of peace, kindness, and radical inclusion. If I am to create my best life, I am to be a person of peace, kindness, and radical inclusion of the beautiful difference that surrounds me, too.

I am far from alone.

The world is filled with fans of Christ who live with a Christlike heart, whether they use the moniker "Christian" or not.

They strive daily to genuinely love their neighbors. Their quest is peaceful and responsible stewardship of people and the earth. They endeavor to walk with the honor of Christ, demonstrating their love for God and Jesus, rejecting the all-consuming and egocentric need to dominate anyone or anything. They don't use the

Religion and Morality Are Not the Same Thing

Bible or their beliefs as a weapon. They appreciate difference, are not hypocrites, and don't stereotype people. These people are not gossips, nor do they denigrate people of other faiths, skin colors, or sexual orientations. They don't listen to or support conspiracy theorists and harbingers of hate or divisiveness. They don't accept hearsay, speculation, or opinion for truth but seek evidence from credible sources before agreeing something or someone is real and truthful. They don't live in fear. They are not consumed by negativity.

I believe what Jesus treasures most about these beautiful friends of his is their hearts, which are filled with empathy, faith, and personal responsibility. They strive each day, no matter how challenging, to behave in alignment with the same values of nonjudgment, compassion, and respect with which Jesus lived.

Sadly, there are also many "Christians" who give Christianity a bad name.

I have encountered Bible teachers who use their positions as a platform to spread their prejudices. I have been spit on, verbally accosted, and physically threatened in the name of God. Sadly, I know many of you have, as well.

Anyone can be dehumanized—LGBTQIA+, people of color, women, the poor, divorced people, nonbelievers, followers of another faith or even just another branch of Christianity. Pseudointellectual talk-show hosts, social-media influencers, television personalities, and celebrity preachers advocate misogyny, racism, homophobia, and anti-immigrant sentiment in their disinformation, false narratives, and infotainment propaganda. These experts of emotional manipulation are supported by millions of Christians who spread their evil as if it were good.

Would Jesus revere people who push blame, divisiveness, and social and religious hate-filled propaganda against those they dehumanize as "other"?

CHAPTER 5

From the very beginning, Christianity has faced internal divisions between those who genuinely strive to live as Jesus did, treating everyone as they want to be treated, and those who want to dominate, control, and dictate the beliefs of other people. We cannot love Jesus and support or turn a blind eye to spiritual frauds who use the religion created in Jesus's honor for ulterior motives. Any attempt to defend negative behavior due to a personal, religious, or political agenda or belief is not aligned with Jesus. Participating in—or even just refusing to condemn—negative behavior is turning our back on Jesus. After all, didn't Jesus remind us, "Truly I say to you, to the extent that you did it to one of these brothers of Mine, even the least of them, you did it to Me" (Matthew 25:40 LSB)?

To be Jesus's friend, we have a duty to stand up against any person, institution, or religious practice that condones or justifies attempts to suppress human rights. The Bible should not be used as a weapon when Jesus himself was an ambassador of love.

Abuses of power are wake-up calls for those who truly admire Christ. For example, I believe Jesus would want all Christians to stand up against those who name themselves as Christian nationalists, who desire to rule over others in his name.

Through their white, male, self-serving interpretation of the Bible, Christian nationalists believe themselves to have a God-given right to rule. They twist Scripture to rationalize their mission of dominance over everyone and everything on earth. Their ideology is fascistic: extremely right-wing, authoritarian, and deeply intolerant of other views or practices.

Christian nationalists willingly shut down the critical reasoning necessary to have a true understanding of what it means to love and follow Jesus, and they reject the message of treating others as they want to be treated. *They have embraced the egocentric*

Religion and Morality Are Not the Same Thing

delusion that to create a path to heaven for themselves, it is acceptable to create a living hell for others.

Activist Reverend Jen Butler observes:

> When you cast God in your own image, you can easily rewrite history with yourself as the hero. Today, people have melted down and recast God in the image of tyrants. Christian Nationalists have cast God as white, male, jingoistic, and American. This God is indistinguishable from the political leaders they swear allegiance to but bears no resemblance to the God of the Bible. . . .
>
> When white Christians are hailed as the heroes, founders, and rightful owners of this country, we deny the full story of the systematic exclusion of people of color, Native Americans, women, LGBTQ+ people, and religious minorities from the benefits of our so-called democracy. This leads to the belief that electing white supremacists "makes America great again" and the belief that elections in which voters of color defeat white supremacists are "stolen elections." Authoritarian rulers perpetuate these lies to exalt themselves and oppress the "other."[14]

Millions of mostly white Americans are hermetically sealed within the ideology of the Christian Right that yearns to destroy the "satanic forces" they blame for the decay of the culture they want to enforce in the country. Ironically, it is our thoughts, words, and actions that create our lives, because God gave us free will. Therefore, the satanic forces we must battle are not outside us but *within our own beliefs* about ourselves and our behavior.

Jesus paid the ultimate price to bring a message of loving compassion to the world. Anyone who desires to rule others in Jesus's

CHAPTER 5

name knows nothing of true sacrifice if the only sacrifice they are willing to embrace is one made by *other* people giving up their rights. But this is the opposite of what Christ taught and how he lived.

Jesus wants us to be courageous in confronting Christian nationalism and other forms of oppression because this evil will not be tamed until it is named and confronted. Christ would not want us to ignore people who cause harm in his name, hoping they will go away. Jesus would challenge us to actively eliminate from Christianity inaccurate versions of what it means to love Christ. For all who say, "I am not one of 'those' Christians"—for people who strive to live authentically with Jesus's empathy and integrity, those who desire truly to follow him—the time has come to rise up and condemn the abuse active within the religion that bears his name.

Doesn't it seem logical that Christianity, as a movement, ought to hold its adherents to the highest standards of Jesus-like integrity rather than excuse corruption, abuse, domination, misinformation, and bigotry?

Does it seem more likely that Jesus expects us to align with people who behave with the same empathy, presence, and integrity he modeled or with those who act otherwise?

Based on everything we know about his example and his message, wouldn't Jesus tell us abuse of power is a great sin—and the abuse of people is just as great?

We don't endear ourselves to Jesus or God by spreading fear and lies about and condemnation of other religions. No matter how many people are fooled into jumping on the bandwagon of fear-based dogma and persecuting people in God's name, Jesus is not fooled. To be right with Jesus, you and I cannot be fooled either because Christianity *has* to inspire us to love one another

Religion and Morality Are Not the Same Thing

as Jesus would. If it cannot, I believe Christ would want his name removed from "Christianity."

To express Jesus's love authentically, we need to push ourselves bravely away from anyone who is comfortable feasting from an all-you-can-eat buffet of fear-based, judgmental, and controlling dogma. These men and women have become numb to the duty they have to Christ to behave with empathy and integrity, as Jesus asks. They simply don't know what they are doing anymore.

Think about this with me for a moment.

Jesus asked God to forgive those who crucified him because they did not know what they were doing; however, this statement implies that their choices—the actions of the heartless and spiritually ignorant—*required forgiveness*. Not praise.

They didn't know what they were doing. But Jesus did. He knew those in the crowd who sold out their integrity and empathy when Pontius Pilate gave them the choice between freeing the criminal Barabbas or him.

And they chose the criminal.

Jesus knew those who tried and executed him were controlled by their egos and their fear.

Just a few days earlier, large crowds had enthusiastically welcomed him. But that was quickly forgotten by those same crowds who, falling victim to groupthink, rationalization, and cognitive dissonance, did an about-face. The crowd was so fearful of admitting their lack of integrity for betraying Jesus that they collectively chose to deny their own recollections of their excitement over his arrival. They went from supporting him to calling for his execution.

Reverends Emily Swan and Ken Wilson write:

CHAPTER 5

The Roman authorities then dressed Jesus (the scapegoat) like a buffoon, with a false crown and purple robe, and beat him until he looked nothing like them. They disfigured, mocked and paraded him around town for all to see, forcing him to carry his own cross until he could carry it no longer. The more different—the more other—he appeared, the easier it would be to dehumanize and kill him. . . .

When Scripture tells us that Jesus bore the sin of the world, he was bearing our projected anxiety, sin and shame. He represented all of the innocent victims—past, present and future—who have ever been excluded, harmed and murdered.[15]

Jesus was despised, rejected, and afflicted. He carried our sorrows. He was wounded for our transgressions. We are part of that crowd. Do we know what we are doing?

How can you and I be sure we are not choosing to side with the criminal(s) again?

Would we stand up for Jesus or fall victim to angry, fearful mob mentality?

Even if *we* don't fully know what we are doing, can we pretend *Jesus* doesn't know the occasions we sell out our empathy and integrity to arrogantly persecute people in his name?

We must remember, too, that *forgiveness does not mean we tolerate abuse*. I am no longer angry with people who despise me for being gay. I forgive them, but I will not permit them to harm me again. I recognize that they are acting out of willful ignorance, steered by fear and groupthink. They don't know me; they only think they do. They don't know what they are doing. I have forgiven them, which, for me, means releasing the ego-motivated resentment I held that kept me an emotional victim of their actions.

Religion and Morality Are Not the Same Thing

Our relationship with Christ and God is personal—a one-on-one experience. We cannot get personal with our spirituality until we invest our heart. We don't invest our heart by allowing our ego to dictate how we treat people. I needed to learn this lesson as much as anyone else. Rather, we choose to act from the soul—the very essence of who we are—as Jesus would. *The bottom line? Being a follower of Christ is much simpler than we make it.*

Jesus asks us to be people of integrity by holding others to the same standards to which we hold ourselves. That's integrity.

Some LGBTQIA+ people behave despicably. So do many straight people.

Some people with dark skin commit crimes. So do many people with light skin.

Human sexuality and skin color don't determine the character values that motivate behavior.

Integrity-focused behavior is governed by the depth of connection we have to the impeccable principles of soul—Jesus's love within our heart. Yes, I am gay and I have shortcomings. Yet as a gay woman who loves Jesus, there is nothing—not money, fame, or power over people—that means more to me than striving to live as Jesus did. Those false measures of success or ways of coping with spiritual emptiness are no longer my idols.

I openly share how I released myself from the grip of my egocentric mind in my book *Lead with Your Heart: Creating a Life of Love, Compassion and Purpose*.[16] I shared openly how I came to terms with my own egocentric decisions and freed myself from such thinking. We all have to be intentional in how we choose to live aligned with Jesus's fundamental definition of success: loving our neighbors as ourselves. Wanting for them what we want for ourselves. Treating all people as we want to be treated. Being responsible stewards of earth and all life. This shouldn't be hard; we already know the standards by which we should operate: ask

CHAPTER 5

what you would want for yourself, and then go and treat other people or the planet the same way.

Of course, no matter how far down the path of spiritual growth we travel, we will never be perfect. But that does not mean we cannot become proficient in walking in the footsteps of Jesus's empathy and integrity. It is the quality of our character that makes us superheroes in Jesus's eyes.

Anyone who says they love Jesus has a duty to honestly answer the question whether Jesus would be proud to call them "friend." People who strive to be proficient in loving as Jesus did don't abuse other people, attempt to control them, work to limit their human rights, or tolerate those who spread hate and divisiveness.

People who genuinely walk alongside Jesus don't deny the fact that he would abhor the idea of White supremacy and giving privilege to an ego-motivated myth that dehumanizes.

People who love Jesus don't turn a blind eye to or perpetuate gender inequity, sexual abuse, or misogyny.

People who care for Jesus don't take a defensive posture when Christianity as a whole is called out for its historical use of fear, discrimination, genocide, slavery, and colonialism as weapons to assert control. The church has justified its actions by insisting it was saving souls, but shouldn't we be asking whether *any* attempt to rationalize dehumanizing people would feel wrong to Jesus's heart?

Pretending our dehumanizing actions don't hurt people would be illogical to Jesus.

In social psychology, cognitive dissonance is the discomfort we feel when we hold conflicting ideas, beliefs, or values at the same time. Because we are uncomfortable, we tend to justify our negative action or belief rather than admit to any wrongdoing.

Religion and Morality Are Not the Same Thing

Like past generations of Christians who enslaved, persecuted, and committed genocide against people in the name of Christ, many who bear the name "Christian" still oppress others under that banner. To love Jesus, and love as Jesus did, we cannot be complicit in accepting judgmental and abusive teachings as God's word or God's will. If we are, we will continue to rely on cognitive dissonance to excuse and justify judgmental, controlling, and cruel behavior.

We must rise like David and defeat the dishonest and dangerous Goliaths of the world. To genuinely love Jesus, we don't treat only those like ourselves well. We treat everyone as we want to be treated. We don't dehumanize others to build up our own power or our sense of "rightness" in the eyes of God. And we certainly don't point to *ourselves* as the victim when someone holds us accountable for our actions.

Anyone, no matter how famous, wealthy, or powerful, who spreads, or refuses to confront those who spread, hate, divisiveness, or abuse of people is a blemish in Jesus's eyes. And if they call themselves Christian, they are a blemish on the religion created in honor of Jesus. If we love Jesus, we can no longer hide from the responsibility we have to Jesus to confront the religious and political abuses we witness, both in ourselves and from other people. What's more, our children learn from watching us and look to us to protect and guide them.

We must show the next generation how to love, and to do that, we must teach them *treating people as we want to be treated does not mean waiting for the other person to go first*. To heal a wounded world, we must lead the way.

That means we act like superheroes and act in bravery. We walk out of any religious service or political rally where leaders or their followers defend the hatred of our human siblings in

CHAPTER 5

the LGBTQIA+ community. Or where they denigrate believers of different religious faiths, women and girls, or those of any other race than their own. Or where they use their influence to press biased political agendas that limit people's human rights. Or where they lie to us, steal from us, or exploit the vulnerable. Or where they don't seem to think it's a problem when someone else does such things.

What if everyone who identifies as Christian (or as a fan of Jesus) courageously moved themselves out of atmospheres of irresponsibility, hate, and disinformation?

What if we bravely challenge the people we entrust with leadership positions?

To trust anyone to help grow our spiritual nature and the sustainability of our world, we need to witness, consistently, that they strive for proficiency in walking in the integrity and empathy of Jesus—with or without the label "Christian."

We don't give power to men and women who ignore their responsibility to be genuine representatives of Jesus's love. We turn away from those who are not willing to hold themselves accountable for the negative influence they have over others. We stand up with Jesus and disassociate ourselves from spiritual frauds. We walk away from toxic teachings and abusive rhetoric. We vigorously refuse to support those who are tarnishing Christ's name. We lead the way in living out the *morality* of our religion, not the malignancy of it.

6

They Are Us and We Are Them

Jesus was Middle Eastern; he had dark skin. Most (if not all) of his earliest followers also had dark skin. And he was a Jew.

According to the beliefs of many people who profess to love and follow Jesus, these attributes should be strikes against him. Why is that?

Fear of difference is deeply rooted in all three Abrahamic religions: Christianity, Judaism, and Islam. (But I'm just here to examine the plank in my own faith's eye.) This was exactly what Jesus was responding to when he challenged the crowds around him to love their neighbors as themselves, but in contemporary Christianity, this fear looks a lot more like viewing anyone or anything different as "the enemy": Protestant versus Catholic, White versus Black and Brown, men versus women, rich versus poor, Republican versus Democrat, conservative versus liberal, heterosexual versus LGBTQIA+, believer versus nonbeliever. The list of "versus" goes on and on. Why do we love our "versus" (and the verses we twist to support each versus) so much when there really is no such thing as "the other"?

One of my most beloved friends, Byll, is over six feet tall and looks like an absolute giant next to his petite wife, Sally, who is

CHAPTER 6

almost five feet. Those of us who know Byll are never surprised when he shows up for a visit wearing a kilt. Sometimes he adds black nail polish to complete an outfit. He has been known to shave his legs for a bike race. Byll loves to defy expectations.

Even though he was accepted to Harvard, he chose to pursue his bachelor's and master of fine arts degrees at a southern college instead. Decades after graduation, he is still continuously learning, devouring books, journal articles, and periodicals on various subjects because he is not a fan of opinion. He is careful to weigh subject matter with great attention to detail, seeking tangible evidence, fact, and public records to shape his views on politics and social justice. He examines the world with an open mind and open heart. He ponders matters so deeply, he could have been Rodin's model for *The Thinker*. And when disagreements arise, he remains even-tempered, respectful, and kind.

Byll is also patient, which is an important merit for our relationship, since I believe in a benevolent, eternal, creative energy I call God, and he does not. This immense difference between us could have ended our friendship before it began, but Byll is a true superhero of integrity who respects me, regardless of how we differ. I respect him too. In fact, our discussions about God challenged me to question why I do believe in God and what I believe God is. Without being urged to examine the rote and often illogical answers programmed into me by my religious upbringing, I almost certainly would not have come to appreciate God as I do now. My atheist friend's calm and peaceful conviction about what is true for *him* helped *me* grow the profound faith I have. With respect as the foundation of our relationship, Byll and I seek to appreciate one another. We approach our friendship with the goal of benefiting from our often divergent beliefs. Both of us want to grasp each other's perspective and engage in discussion

They Are Us and We Are Them

about it. Engaging with each other in this way is not easy, but it is rewarding and enlightening.

Have you ever discussed God with an atheist or scientist? To understand one another, we have to stop assuming shared beliefs are a prerequisite for respect and relationship. Doesn't it seem as if Jesus would encourage us to listen and attempt to comprehend other people and their viewpoints rather than just rejecting them outright?

Jesus led with his soul and his heart—with wisdom, compassion, and enlightenment. God created us souls so we, too, can lead with the higher, wiser, loving part of ourselves. When we don't, ego takes control. And ego's arrogant need for people to support our viewpoints or to make ourselves right and other people wrong is insatiable. How is ego's condemnation of the "other" aligned with our loving soul's appreciation of creation?

My atheist friend Byll is one of the kindest people I have ever met. I know from years of observing him model a deep reverence for people, and all life, his actions are not dependent upon a belief in God or devotion to the Bible or any religious identity, but they are every bit as genuine and heartfelt as my own efforts in this area. Neither of us is perfect. But striving to live as love in action is our shared goal. Even if I am the only one who believes that living in love is to honor Jesus, we both do it because, as both atheist and believer, we agree there is no room for unhealthy ego in healthy relationships.

Whether we are believers or not, who we are is evident by how we treat ourselves and other people. To love my friend as Jesus would, I don't judge Byll's absence of belief in God. If I were to attempt to love my friend with my ego, I would argue with him and try to convert him. Frustration, fear, and attempts to convert him would all be egotistical, even when my ego would attempt

CHAPTER 6

to rationalize that I am doing God's work. We can commit to calmly standing firm in our beliefs without having to convince, dictate, or force anyone to believe as we do. And we can accept that to believe or not is a part of the power of responsible choice God put into each heart.

Please know I mean no disrespect to anyone, and certainly not to God, but when we consider it logically and lovingly, can we honestly say God cares whether we believe in God or not? Doesn't the idea that God demands for us to believe mean God is conceited and prideful? Yet God is neither conceited nor prideful, as God has no ego. Even in human form, God-as-Jesus emptied himself of ego during the forty days he was in the desert wrestling with temptation. Jesus was battling his human, dark side—the anger, bitterness, and blame—to live from his fearless, loving, divine soul.

Ego does not do God's work. It is only with the integrity of humility that we can learn to master our self-righteous ego in order live from our soul. We volunteer to do this personal assessment to honor Jesus, as we are charged by God to live as Jesus did, following the only dogmas ever needed: love and kindness.

His Holiness the fourteenth Dalai Lama Tenzin Gyatso once said, "My true religion, my simple faith is in love and compassion. There is no need for complicated philosophy, doctrine, or dogma. Our own heart, our own mind, is the temple. The doctrine is compassion. Love for others and respect for their rights and dignity, no matter who or what they are—these are ultimately all we need."[17] How very Christlike for the Dalai Lama, a Tibetan Buddhist, to promote the uncomplicated goal of living with integrity as love in action. And yet, when I posted this quote on social media, I received several messages chastising me with, "A true Christian would never promote another religion."

They Are Us and We Are Them

Instead of striving to lead with acceptance and love of heart, as Christ lived, many of us use our beliefs to wage religious battles against other faiths, against other branches within our own faith, and sometimes even against everyone else except our own narrow brand of "Christian."

Jesus would remind us we are all supposed to be on the same team. But, heartbreakingly, many people who claim to follow him seem to have no desire for that. How can we create the peaceful and compassionate world Jesus envisioned for us as long as spirituality is viewed as a zero-sum game?

Brought up in a fundamentalist church, I was exposed to a condescending, holier-than-thou attitude from the beginning. This arrogance on the part of those who claimed to love Jesus—and their blatant condemnation of people in Jesus's name—eventually led me to understand my religious experience as one of narrow-minded human beings attempting to keep an infinite God in a box of limited conception.

They wanted to control ideas about God and other people. Doing so made them feel better about life and better than other people—which, by their reckoning, appeared to mean they had the right to force people to adopt the same beliefs they held or to persecute them as sinners.

Ego's perceived superiority rationalizes the attempt to win people to our point of view as caring for one another's spiritual salvation—no matter how twisted or cruel that may be. This is ironic, given that arrogance, blame, and abuse of people in God's name should be unacceptable to our souls. Leading with ego's superiority is not how Christ guided us to approach life. He was peaceful and humble. He wanted to know why people thought as they did. Christ showed us the importance of evaluating people's behavior to determine their personal integrity through their

CHAPTER 6

accountability, respect, and civility. But as soon as we persecute someone who does not view God as we believe they should or exist in the world according to the artificial standards we have set, we have fallen victim to our human ego's arrogance.

Arrogance stops us from listening to and appreciating different viewpoints and experiences. When ego controls us, we are certain our beliefs are the only ones worth having, even when the beliefs we hold are controlling and injurious to people. With conceit in charge of our attitudes, we don't see the need to even challenge our beliefs. With ego in control, we are tempted to follow the practice of thinking or making decisions as a group. When we allow groupthink to guide us, we discourage creativity and individual responsibility. And ego will maintain an irrational loyalty to what we want to believe, even when we witness unloving, corrupt, or evil behavior in ourselves and other people. Our ego's superiority is quick to blind us to our flaws.

Ego will certainly not voluntarily admit our wrongdoings. Ego wants only to view itself as right, better, and smarter, and it even judges itself to be kinder and more loving than others, even when our behavior is actually the opposite.

For lovers of Jesus, it is important to acknowledge an arrogant attitude does not originate from our spiritual side, even when our egotism convinces us we are obeying God's word or doing God's work. Ego's haughtiness is condescending and sarcastic—"God made Adam and Eve, not Adam and Steve." "Love the sinner but hate the sin." Ego loves pithy zingers but hates to be challenged in any depth.

It is not God's will but human judgment that seeks to put someone else "in their place." God only cares whether we behave as the eternal soul we are, an ambassador of love who treats all people and life as we want to be treated. And following the

They Are Us and We Are Them

Golden Rule means we do the right thing, even when other people choose not to.

I was standing alone at the bus stop when a woman carrying a Bible came up to me, pointed at my Romancing Your Soul shoulder bag, and said, "You're a witch. That's the devil's work. Only if Jesus is your Lord will you be saved."

I smiled at her and stayed silent. She turned and walked away.

After years of wrestling with my own understanding about who or what God is, I now accept God as loving. Just that: loving. Regardless of how I am treated or what I am accused of, unless I am physically in danger, I will do my very best to express myself as love—through kindness, respect, and forgiveness. For me, being love in action is what the God I believe in desires each of us to strive for.

Our soul is the eternal part of our being, where the values of integrity and empathy reside. And the home to our eternal soul is a human body with a personality and ego. A healthy ego, or sense of self, allows us to see ourselves in one another, to consider the needs, thoughts, and desires of others. With a healthy ego, we can see the big picture and how all life is connected. We understand and care about how the actions we take today will affect the world for our children and their children. When we are guided by healthy self-esteem, we welcome constructive criticism and accept responsibility for our thoughts, words, and the consequences of our actions. We desire to learn from the experience and observations of other people, from our history, and from our own choices (both positive and negative). A healthy, balanced sense of self depends on the moral and ethical integrity of soul to guide our behavior.

However, when our ego is unhealthy, we discount the ethical and moral part of ourselves and others. A self-absorbed ego is fo-

CHAPTER 6

cused on satisfying its unending lust for immediate gratification, power, and control and will vilify and blame anyone who gets in its way. An overinflated sense of self will justify any behavior in order for us to get what we want, when and how we want it. Unhealthy ego has no problem lying about anything to anyone and is very skilled at getting people to believe the lies we tell. Left unchecked, the ego's arrogance, irresponsibility, and contempt can eventually destroy us, our relationships, and our world.

We have to appreciate that walking in Jesus's footsteps may be simple but requires deliberate effort. Perhaps we should dedicate more religious attention to how we can overrule unhealthy human ego to lead with divine love. God gave you and me a soul so we can care for one another as Jesus cares for us. And we have to choose to lead with the higher, wiser, logical, and loving part of ourselves because we don't love with our ego.

Ego's ignorance will not admit it is ignorant. Ego's stupidity will not admit it is reckless. Ego's jealousy and envy will not acknowledge it is jealous or envious. Ego will always place blame elsewhere. Ego will always defend itself. Ego is impatient and unconscious to our actions. Ego relies on easy labels rather than nuanced thinking to make sense of other people and to secure one's own feelings of security and "rightness."

In order to love as Jesus did, we choose to look beyond one-dimensional labels that don't mean anything to God. After all, if the goal of lovers of Christ is to live an egoless life as Jesus did, why do we live in fear of difference, of losing control, or of the unknowable?

No matter the skin color, gender, or sexuality of our human body, the integrity of our soul matters most to God, so it should matter the most to us as well. Since soul is home to the honesty,

They Are Us and We Are Them

empathy, and respect of our integrity, we can only love one another as, and with, souls.

At my local pharmacy, there is a kind, joyful, and respectful Muslim woman who wears a hijab. Each time I go into the store, she smiles as she waits on customers. She treats each person with warmth and kindness, as she would a friend.

This woman's behavior represents the best of her religious beliefs. Certainly not all Muslims behave as she does, just as all Christians don't behave in alignment with Jesus.

Religious labels don't make us God's chosen people. God cares that we do everything in our power to live each day as an ambassador of love by mastering haughty self-centeredness to live from humble soul.

We master our egocentric side by wanting to do so. We acknowledge our self-centered, jealous, envious side, and then we work purposefully to remain present with our thoughts and behavior to transform an unhealthy sense of self into healthy self-esteem and self-respect. We determine our own personal worth by the way we honor God by showing respect to ourselves, to other people, and to all life.

We work each day to be more respectful and inclusive of difference than we were yesterday. We look for integrity and empathy in people, and we work to overcome selfishness in order to live in line with Christ's selfless love. This is the way—the only way—we can be a superhero for Jesus.

7

Sometimes We Turn the Other Cheek and Other Times We Don't

Why does it seem so difficult to know when to turn the other cheek and when not to?

We know unhealthy ego wants us to fight fire with fire. But it is our soul—our heart connection to a wise and loving God—that can determine when it is best to cool a heated situation and when it is best to tackle abuse and injustice head-on.

I was the only person waiting in line one day at a coffee shop when a man entered the store and approached the counter. At first I thought he had not seen me standing in line, so I said, "Sir, the line starts over here."

He looked at me and said, "You can wait. I am in a hurry." Then he placed his order.

I know what you're probably thinking. My pride reactively thought the same things: *How dare he act so rudely? Who does he think he is? How can anyone behave with such calloused entitlement and disrespect? Someone ought to teach him a lesson!*

But . . .

Doesn't the universal spiritual message and standard to guide our daily behavior—the Golden Rule—emphasize treating peo-

Sometimes We Turn the Other Cheek and Other Times We Don't

ple as we want to be treated . . . *even if they behave in self-centered and rude ways that cause us to want to call them an asshole?*

There was a time in my life when I would have continued engaging with the self-centered man or implored management to intervene in an attempt to get him to apologize. However, I have learned the benefit of not reacting or stooping to the same level of awareness (or unawareness, in this case) that creates a negative situation in the first place.

I did not know the man. So I let the "nonviolent" actions of the ill-mannered stranger go.

There is no winner in an ego-boxing match, and Jesus encourages us to pick our battles.

The soul wisdom of knowing when it is best to turn the other cheek to someone's entitled and irresponsible side was hard-won for me.

If a stranger was rude, I relished calling them on their unconscious behavior. If an inconsiderate driver cut me off, I freely gave them the middle finger. If a man verbally assaulted me with homophobic slurs, I happily insulted his manhood.

I perfected the art of ego boxing with rude, callous individuals before I woke up to the futility of fighting someone's self-centeredness with my own ego's arrogance. Never once did someone I chastised or insulted acknowledge their behavior. Not one time did anyone express appreciation to me for helping wake them up to their unacceptable actions. Ego simply wants to do battle rather than assume responsibility for how we behave. These individuals believed they were entitled to their rude, arrogant, or ignorant choices, and I believed I was entitled to respond in kind. In each case, we both believed our desires were more important than the other person's, so we were never going to back down.

CHAPTER 7

This is the exact same rationale that leads to companies firing whistleblowers. When confronted about their illegal or unethical actions people in positions of power alter evidence, manufacture false information, or lie in an attempt to shift blame from themselves. They work to ruin the reputation of the brave individual who confronted them rather than assume responsibility for their actions.

Ego does not like to be confronted. It protects itself. We lie, for instance, and our ego then creates a web of lies in a desperate attempt to get away with the first lie. And that creates a "big" lie.

Unless we love and respect ourselves by controlling our own arrogant, defensive, and unkind side, we will readily abandon our integrity and empathy—as well as our call to love and respect others. This requires us to weigh the situations we find ourselves in from Christ's perspective. Christ *did not* always turn the other cheek; he called out injustice and abuse. But he carefully led with his soul to determine which battles to wage. To be a true friend of Jesus, we need to do the same.

I imagine the times Jesus turned the other cheek were the occasions when he knew it would be impossible to reason with an unreasonable person. He knew it would be pointless to engage with someone who was consumed by their arrogant and controlling side.

I think it's safe to say Jesus would not have ego boxed with social-media trolls.

We also know he was a teacher; in fact, he is called "teacher" forty-five times across the Four Gospels. The point of teaching is to leave the student somehow changed for the better; therefore, Jesus probably would not want me to scream at the guy in the coffee shop—no matter how much I may want to—because lowering ourselves to the irresponsible behavior of egotistical people does not change us for the better.

Sometimes We Turn the Other Cheek and Other Times We Don't

In these types of irritating (but not dangerous) situations, it seems reasonable to assume Jesus would ask us to turn the other cheek. We take a few deep breaths and stop ourselves from reacting with ego. We appreciate not all of us are on the same level of measuring our thoughts, words, and actions against a courteous and responsible standard of behavior.

I am certain many people in Jesus's time thought him weak when he chose to turn the other cheek. Likewise, there may be some who consider us weak, too, for not engaging with people like a rude driver or the man in the coffee shop. I believe in these cases we become the stronger party for having the ability to control ourselves.

That doesn't mean we stay silent; I did offer the man the opportunity to correct his behavior. He had the opportunity to do the right thing. He chose not to. I chose to turn the other cheek in this instance because, ultimately, *we are not responsible for how people choose to behave.*

Several years ago, one of the most important people in my life, my aunt, passed away in a Texas hospital at the age of ninety-two. The entire week leading up to her death was an extraordinarily stressful and exhausting experience. I returned to the hotel each evening drained.

Just before midnight on the same day we lost my aunt, a large group of college students arrived at the hotel. They yelled to one another as they got off the elevators. They slammed doors. It was the middle of the night in a crowded hotel, and yet they carried on for over an hour, oblivious to anyone other than themselves.

The next morning I got on an elevator with several of the young people just in time to hear the group openly insulting gay people and people of color. They wore name tags and crosses and had on Christian T-shirts; it turned out they were there for a spiritual retreat.

CHAPTER 7

You can imagine how my ego was screaming for me to say something witty and profound. Ego wanted me to block the elevator doors and give them an hour-long sermon on what I believe it means to love and follow Jesus. But I thought of Jesus and how he would respond and stayed silent, even while my mind swirled with questions:

> *Do we think Jesus would be okay with excusing their inconsiderate actions and intolerance as "just kids being kids"?*
> *Don't homophobic, inconsiderate, and bigoted children grow into homophobic, inconsiderate, and bigoted adults?*
> *Why do any of our young people believe persecution and self-centeredness are acceptable behavior?*
> *Whom did they learn this behavior from? Religious leaders, their parents, their peers? Did they learn it on social media or in their Christian colleges?*
> *Isn't it an appropriate undertaking to teach children how to be responsible representatives of Jesus?*

I know how difficult a task staying silent can be. And I also know when people are confronted with how they are behaving, ego is quick to defend their actions or to cast blame elsewhere. Groupthink is a powerful thing and often leads to aggression and even violence against those who go against the crowd—which I know from experience is painfully true.

Standing in that elevator, debating whether to speak up, I was reminded of a time when I, too, went on a Christian youth retreat. While on a walk, a group of us came to a small house sitting all alone in the middle of a big forest. Curiosity overruled the respect we should have had for private property. Our group went inside the unlocked home and some of the kids started vandalizing it for fun. I left, not wanting to take part.

Sometimes We Turn the Other Cheek and Other Times We Don't

Later that day a man appeared at the retreat camp and engaged in a heated discussion with the adult retreat leaders. After he left they rang a dinner bell to gather everyone and insisted we tell them what we knew.

Silence fell over the group. No one spoke up as I sat, fighting with my conscience over whether to do what I had been told was right—what Jesus would do—and be honest, or to protect myself by keeping silent, not wanting to be labeled a snitch. Yet, I knew Jesus did not turn the other cheek when harm was done to innocent parties.

After what seemed an unbearable length of time, I spoke up. By confessing, I intentionally chose to overrule my irresponsible ego in order to live from responsible soul. While many of us have been indoctrinated to observe a culture of politeness and loyalty over honesty, we don't remain silent about everything. In that instance, I chose not to fall in line and maintain a culture of not rocking the boat. These were not strangers in a coffee shop or on an elevator who inconvenienced or disrespected me. These were my friends, my brothers and sisters in Christ, who had caused injury to someone else.

I will never forget the hateful looks I got from many of those kids. Not one of the guilty people confessed. No one spoke up to defend or confirm my story. Their terrible stares told me there would be hell to pay for being honest.

After supper that night a group of the guilty kids dragged me out of my cabin when I was alone. They covered me in shaving cream and rolled me in the dirt and leaves. They pulled me around by my arms. Sticks and rocks cut into my body. The shaving cream burned my eyes.

They did not care about doing what Jesus would do. Instead, as a group, they justified treating me cruelly because they agreed it was an appropriate punishment for speaking against the group.

CHAPTER 7

My friends made me the scapegoat for their crimes that day. As soon as I told the truth, those young people collectively viewed themselves as victims. Then, as a mob, they justified making me the guilty one—the "other." Throughout my life there have been times when I went along with the crowd, too, and betrayed an innocent person. I did not want to be singled out, so I shoved aside my integrity in favor of public approval. In doing so, I betrayed not only myself and the innocent person but also Jesus—someone who knows all too well what it means to be scapegoated by a mob.

All of this was going through my mind as I rode that elevator with those college kids, thirty years later. We reached the lobby, the doors opened, and I exited without saying a word.

Reverends Emily Swan and Ken Wilson write:

> In a sense, our worst—our distinctly human—crime is this: fueled by mimetic desire, we resolve our internal group conflicts (in families, on the job, in society) by targeting a vulnerable member or minority group. We accuse them of faults we are blind to in ourselves, projecting onto them what we are loath to face in ourselves. As we write this, the "scapegoats du jour" include Muslims, immigrants, global financiers (code for the Jews), advocates of Black Lives Matter, members of the "dishonest" press—always, there is some "other" causing our problems. We stigmatize, isolate, silence and oppress "those people" . . . and it brings a temporary sense of unity to the crowd organizing itself around these accusations. We resort to this mechanism again and again, forever blind to the innocence of those we target—the guilty ones who are, in fact, the objects of our own projected guilt. Scapegoating is "that thing we do." And the way to undo it is to unmask it.[18]

Sometimes We Turn the Other Cheek and Other Times We Don't

To love and follow Jesus, we must honestly ask ourselves: *How often do we allow ego to blame our shortcomings and irresponsibility on others because we choose not to behave responsibly, no matter the outcome?*

The mastery of ego is a continuous, moment-by-moment devotion to integrity we undertake for the rest of our lives. It is a daily Inipi ceremony in which endless challenges arise. We don't master a mind that has a mind of its own (ego) just once and then we are done. Our egocentric mind continuously thinks about ways to justify our actions or validate our fears and beliefs and will continue to do so until we pass away.

Our ego's tendency to escape responsibility is why we have to honestly and enduringly love Jesus and ourselves by caring that there are consequences to all behavior. We love Jesus by being devoted to the moment-by-moment duty of evaluating our attitudes and behavior and assessing our relationship to the behavior and attitudes of others, including those who say they love Jesus. After all, *why say we want to follow Jesus if we're not dedicated to walking in his footsteps—both when he acted and when he refrained from acting?*

We are obliged to live an honest life. We want to learn from the irresponsible choices we make so we can do better the next time we face a similar situation. We own our behavior because in order to grow our loving nature, we must have spiritual awareness. As C. S. Lewis observed, "Evil comes from the abuse of free will. . . . Why, then, did God give us free will? Because free will, though it makes evil possible, is also the only thing that makes possible any love or goodness or joy worth having."[19]

I began smoking when I was in my twenties. For the next twenty-two years, I was addicted. Some days I smoked two packs. It was like setting money on fire, not to mention the constant cough-

CHAPTER 7

ing, bad breath, horrible-smelling clothing, recurring bronchitis, and inability to walk up a flight of stairs without having to rest.

By the time I was in my early thirties, I was terrified of dying. Yet day after day, year after year, I continued to justify smoking. It was one way I chose to stuff down my emotional pain. With each inhale, I sucked in more self-hatred, denial, and disappointment. Even though I detested being under the control of a tiny white tube of tobacco, my mind told me I was too weak-willed to quit. The fear and justification created by my mind, which had a stubborn and illogical logic of its own, halted even the slightest movement forward. I kept turning my gaze away from the truth of my situation.

Until one day, out of the blue, the truth hit me. I wasn't weak; I was strong for having survived all of the challenges and heartbreak life had thrown at me. I was just scared of what life would be like and who I would be without the emotional crutch I had used to mask my fear for more than two decades.

The game-changing moment came when I finally had the courage to look honestly at the reason I was using cigarettes: to avoid opening up to loving and respecting myself. And I realized no matter how painful life had been, continuing to hurt myself was even more painful and disappointing. Hurting myself would never get back at the people who had hurt me.

Overcoming our fearful ego requires moving from a victim's perspective to a victor's. Even if we truly were victims, we love ourselves by exercising God's gift of purposeful choice to create responsible lives. We acknowledge *we* are the ones in control of our actions. There is no outside influence that controls our behavior. Wouldn't Jesus want us to stop and consider which side of ourselves, ego or soul, we are about to present before we speak or act? To know when to speak up and when to stay silent, we control

Sometimes We Turn the Other Cheek and Other Times We Don't

our ego and exercise God's gift of responsible choice over our behavior. Only our logical, responsible, and loving soul chooses the right battles to wage in Jesus's name by knowing when to turn the other cheek and when not to.

Since we cannot control or change anyone but ourselves, we must rise above and win the battle over ego and behave with integrity from our very soul. Put another way, "Do not be overcome by evil, but overcome evil with good" (Romans 12:21).

8

Men of Quality Respect Women's Equality

Pop quiz: which Marvel Comics Avenger superhero do you think is considered the strongest?
Iron Man, Thor, or Hulk?
Doctor Strange, Nick Fury, or Spider Man?
Winter Soldier, Captain America, or Black Panther?
Well, if you chose any of these, you'd be wrong—at least according to writer and superhero superfan Kyshaun Drakes. He ranks the top Avengers in the Marvel Cinematic Universe (MCU) in his article "MCU: The Strongest and Weakest Members of the Avengers." And coming in on top is not a hero at all but a heroine—Scarlet Witch/Wanda Maximoff.[20]

Even though these are just fantasy superheroes, Drakes's ranking sets a positive example. When a man values a woman's strength, he respects her personal freedom, individuality, and ambitions as if they were his own.

This is something a real-life superhero man of quality taught me.

I was in my late thirties when my atheist friend Byll and his wife, Sally, moved in next door. Over the next seven years, Byll became my best friend. Even though he did not believe in God, Byll was gentler, more respectful, and more supportive than any man in my life who had professed to be God-loving had ever been.

In his presence, it felt safe for me to confront the pain and anger of being born a gay woman in a male-dominated world filled with religiously justified misogyny, inequity, and abuse. The marathon hours we spent talking and sharing slowly opened my heart. I began healing a deeply wounded sense of unworthiness, shame, and inadequacy. Byll taught me intimacy has nothing to do with sex and everything to do with honestly baring your soul to another who holds it safe.

I believe God has a sense of humor, given that it took finding deep friendship with a man for this gay and oppressed woman to open her heart to men and to God. Byll encouraged me to question the motives behind all religions, societies, and political parties that suppress, subjugate, or attempt to control women. Together, we questioned why we as a human society continue to turn the other cheek to sexual abuse, gender inequity, and male domination of females—why we continue to prop up the patriarchy.

John Zerzan states the danger of continued inequity between genders: "Civilization, very fundamentally, is the patriarchal history of the domination of nature and of the rule over women. What a sad but true legacy we are leaving to our children and theirs. We cannot expect our children to have balanced and peaceful relationships while continuing to teach girls they are less than boys. We cannot expect boys to grow into loving and respectful men if we place them more important than women."[21]

For thousands of years, society has passed along ancient religious and cultural beliefs that support and perpetuate vast gender inequity of power by favoring men, resulting in continuous economic, social, and political injustice for women. The ongoing

CHAPTER 8

disdain for women and belittlement of the values commonly associated with the feminine have a well-established history in our world religions. Leonard Shlain observes: "The history of Christianity, Islam and Taoism darkly demonstrates that the religions that flowed from the teachings of Jesus, Muhammad and Lao Tzu have been most unkind to women. In every case, after the death of the founder, men with harsh patriarchal leanings seized the reins of power and revised whatever gentle counsel the originators of these traditions may have had to impart about women."[22]

Fast forward two thousand years from Christ's death, and women still don't have safety from sexual abuse, equity within Western society and the church, or the respect Christ afforded women millennia ago.

Why is that?

We continue to subscribe to male-dominated societies that today, both subtly and overtly, promote the patriarchal philosophy that men are superior and women are inferior. Ancient and controlling religious beliefs remain steeped in male-controlled traditions where women are indoctrinated to be subservient.

My almost-one-hundred-year-old mother had a conversation with a woman who, without remorse, said, "Women will never have any power or say in my Baptist church, and that is exactly how God wants it."

A Roman Catholic woman responded to my post on social media about the importance of gender equity by writing, "Women are to be subservient. We may not like it but that is just the way it is and has to be. After all it was Eve who committed the original sin."

A conservative Catholic woman on the highest court in the nation disregards the personal liberties of all women to make their own health-care choices regarding abortion (even in the

Men of Quality Respect Women's Equality

cases of rape and incest). Her reasoning is her religious belief that a fertilized egg is a human being—even though neither Jesus nor the Bible ever said any such thing.

It is important for you and me to understand that if people appointed to the Supreme Court, the Fifth Circuit Court,[23] or any court are to protect the rights of all citizens from a tyranny of a minority, they should not be politically biased in any way, such as the opinion espoused by the Federalist Society and their billionaire backers that the US Constitution is an unchanging document. This is important to know, since six of the current nine Justices of the Supreme Court, all appointed by Republican Presidents, are, or were, members of the Federalist Society.[24]

To believe the Constitution is a set-in-stone, unchanging document is similar to the belief that the Bible is the infallible word of God, with no regard for cultural or historical context. Likewise, male, White, Eurocentric scholarship has dominated biblical interpretation for the past several centuries. Harvard-educated legal scholar and author of *Allow Me to Retort: A Black Guy's Guide to the Constitution* Elie Mystal conveyed in an interview,

> We have been told a lot by Conservative White people what the Constitution means, what the law means, how it should be interpreted and why. And that, from my perspective, is just one option among many. The other options involve looking at the Constitution as a flawed document that needs to be perfected in order to achieve a level of fundamental fairness and equality that was, shall we say, missing from the initial draft of it, [a draft that was] written by slavers, colonists, and people willing to make deals with slavers and colonists.
>
> Do you want to know why the Constitution doesn't explicitly protect a woman's right to choose? Because the Con-

CHAPTER 8

stitution did not explicitly protect a woman's right to talk, or to own property, or to not be raped. There's a lot of things that the Constitution doesn't protect when it comes to the issue of women's rights, because the Constitution did not treat women as full people.[25]

Mystal goes on to point out that not only were women excluded from writing the Constitution back in the 1780s but no woman has ever helped to write any of the twenty-seven amendments that currently exist. (It's true! Look it up.) Women have never made up a majority of the Supreme Court, either. Mystal asserts that in order for the Constitution to have any relevance as a legally binding document intended to ensure and protect the rights of all citizens of the United States, "it must evolve, it must breathe, it must live in a world where we understand the rights and responsibilities in this country a little bit more expansively than the exclusively White cis-hetero men that have been allowed to adjudicate those rights for most of our history."[26]

Patriarchal societies cannot solve the problem of gender inequity while continuing to uphold gender inequality. And what society is more patriarchal in the Western world than the church? To move ourselves forward, we consider that the true original sin had nothing to do with a woman taking fruit and everything to do with men taking away women's agency in the name of God—the belief (perpetuated by male authors of the Bible) that Eve was less than Adam and, by extension, that women and girls are something to control and dominate.

As a teenager, I was instructed to lose at sports on purpose because when I consistently won, many of my male playmates were furious.

Men of Quality Respect Women's Equality

Even when my experience and education level were often the same as or greater than theirs, my male coworkers consistently made more money than I did. And still do.

When men or boys speak up against perceived injustice, they are applauded. When I do, I am labeled a bitch.

In the words of Shirley Anita Chisholm, American politician, educator, and author, "The emotional, sexual, and psychological stereotyping of females begins when the doctor says: 'It is a girl.'"[27]

So let's ask ourselves:

> Women, how old were you when you began to notice you were considered less than your male counterparts? (I was in early elementary school when this reality hit me.)
>
> Men, how old were you when you began to understand you were considered more important than women and girls? (My friend Leslie was around eleven when he began realizing there were differences in the way society treated boys and girls and that he was regarded as more important because he was a boy.)

Both within the church and outside of it, both intentionally and due to unconscious bias, girls and boys alike learn that one of them is "better" than the other. We shouldn't even have to ask the question, and yet, here we are: *How is it logical to believe God is gender-biased when Jesus was an advocate for women as his equals?*

Jesus honored and respected women. Women were valued members of his inner circle. Religious scholars believe women were among his disciples. Jesus was not threatened by women and, therefore, did not desire to control or dominate them. He did not view women as servants to men or as sexual objects or as weaker, less intelligent, or incapable of contributing equally to spirituality or society. Surely such a man would not value women based solely on their appearance, sweetness, submissiveness, or sexual availability.

For our modern civilization to thrive, or even survive, I believe one of the most important challenges we face is that of putting an end to gender inequity and abuse against women, acts that are perpetuated by ancient patriarchal religious and social beliefs about male power.

But how?

By evolving the inaccurate and harmful patriarchal mindset to instead embrace Genesis 1:27, which states every person is created *b'tzelem Elohim*—"in God's image." Our own Bible tells us that every person is equally important and has infinite potential to make a unique, positive contribution in the world. Doesn't it make sense that if a supreme awareness initiated the creation of everything, then that consciousness resides in every person in equal measure?

To view women and men as equal, we need to grow our spiritual consciousness by awakening to the truth that patriarchal societies were created and are sustained, in part, by the concept of a male God.

Gender inequity, abuse, and the suppression of women are in part rooted in the continued religious labeling of the supreme consciousness as male. As feminist scholar Mary Daly famously wrote, "If God is male, then male is God."[28]

Even my atheist friend Byll agreed if there is a God, that God is too expansive to be labeled or fit into a specific gender. However, in the Christian church (and several other world religions), we are taught God is male. Yet wouldn't it be logical and loving to question whether the message of God as male motivates many men to believe they are entitled to treat women as less than themselves? Shouldn't we at least explore the possibility that somewhere along the line, religious men with a very specific agenda took pains to create God in *their own image*? I don't mean addressing God in the gendered term "Father"; that's a beautiful image of a protecting and loving parent. I mean the portrayal of God as utterly and only male. If tradition-bound religious leaders don't actually believe women are inherently less than men (as many of them claim), just watch how they react if you dare to address God as "Mother."

These are timely and important questions. Our minds use labels to separate, elevate, and judge. Gay, Black, woman. As soon as a label is placed on something or someone, our mind's arrogance latches on. Conceit blinds us to other possibilities, even when faced with the truth that belief in God as male helps, in both overt and subtle ways, to perpetuate the social, sexual, and economic abuse of power over women.

When a man takes charge, he has leadership capabilities. When a woman takes charge, she's bossy or a "bitch."

When men share news about people, they are "shooting the breeze." When women do the same, they are gossiping.

For men to get angry is acceptable. But if a woman gets just as angry, she is labeled "crazy."

When a woman disagrees with a man, she's threatening. When a man disagrees with another man, it's nonthreatening.

Women are labeled fat but men simply have "love handles."

When a boy attracts girls, he's popular. When a girl attracts the opposite sex, she's a flirt.

A woman gets pregnant and it's her fault. Yet where's the logic of not making the owner of the penis equally responsible?

Although it may be easy for people to dismiss me as an angry woman for shining light on the double standards created in part by continuing to label God male, my doing so comes from a place of deep respect for both women and men. And for God.

CHAPTER 8

I realize we can continue to debate this with our egos. But if we use our hearts, the souls we are that have no gender, we have to admit an inclusive Jesus would never condone abuse or female suppression.

So let's imagine an all-embracing Jesus would ask us to move our collective spiritual consciousness forward in this way: *Just call God "God," without assigning a gender.* If it is hard to wrap our minds around this because of male-dominated religious indoctrination, then I believe Jesus would want us to honestly ask, with our hearts:

How can God be exclusively male when life is birthed from female?
Wouldn't thinking of God as both female and male be a positive step toward establishing gender equity?
Or what if we humbly view God as being without human form?

There are many Christians, as well as people of other religious faiths, who value a female/male or genderless view of God. Among them is my friend Caleb, who finds this view of God to be a positive addition to his relationships, his self-image, and his spirituality. In his words communicated to me by email on June 5, 2019, he said:

> We play somewhat traditional roles in our family. I work and my wife is a full-time mom. My job is easier, but I didn't always feel that way. I spent the first several years of our marriage pursuing a career in acting and operating my own business. It was wonderful and afforded me the opportunity to be at home rather than in an office. As our children were born, instead of meetings and business trips, I found myself washing out bottles, changing diapers, helping out with twi-

Men of Quality Respect Women's Equality

light feedings, and sharing in the household responsibilities of keeping our home clean and organized.

Initially my ego resisted these experiences. "What am I doing this for? I need to be out earning more money. I just cleaned this up, I shouldn't have to again. I don't feel like going to the grocery store for baby food right now!"

Slowly I began to take responsibility for these "chores" and realized they were privileges. God lavished me with the blessings of a wonderful marriage and two precious children. I washed our dishes not because I was nagged to do it, but because they were our dishes and they needed to be cleaned. My wife always championed my efforts and expressed constantly how much she appreciated my help and how much it meant to her. That made me feel ten feet tall. I learned I didn't need a boardroom and a million dollars to be a husband. I could simply love my wife and show her my support by helping out around our home, and that was enough. This helped me discover value in the nurturing, sensitive, feminine side of my personality and it changed the way I approached the more "masculine" duties I also had. Helping with our family removed a significant amount of ego and showed me that the two separate worlds of male/female I saw growing up should overlap.

It is challenging these days to hold binary views of gender-specific roles, and that is a good thing. I believe both men and women were created in the image of God. I believe God is love. Love so pure and powerful that it transcends our human understanding of sexual gender. I have felt a strong masculine love from God. It has brought me strength, provided direction, and protected me. I have also felt an equally strong feminine love from God. A motherly love that has

CHAPTER 8

brought me comfort, held me like a child, provided wisdom and understanding with a gentleness that can only be described as Divine. With this dual context of God's love, we now have a different lens to view not only God's love, but how we reflect God's love with each other.

Jesus would want us all to embrace the fact that God made all human beings, which means we are obliged to respect one another equally as God's children. To do so we must honor God and move Christianity away from a patriarchal view of a male God to focus on the fact that *Jesus was an example of how empowered men are to empower women.*

Jesus respected women. He honored them. He valued them. Christ viewed women as his equals, and I seriously doubt he was single. According to Jewish law and customs of the day, girls were usually engaged sometime between the ages of twelve and fifteen and would be married at around fifteen or sixteen. Boys would have been married by around nineteen or twenty years of age. Religious scholars now speculate Jesus was married with children.

Honestly, *wouldn't Jesus being married with a family make him more relatable?*

Again, our faith in God is not in peril if we question the Bible, or that God is male, or that Jesus was also human like us. The fact is, we don't know whether Jesus was married. In the Bible, we learn only what male scribes transcribed from oral tradition. Religious scholars caution that the men who wrote the Bible often did so with bias, going so far as to reflect ancient beliefs about gender roles or to translate the Bible in ways to reflect the desires of the rulers of the period in which they lived. For example, the King James Version of the Bible was translated specifically to ensure it would conform to the beliefs of the church and of the ordained White, male clergy, all of whom were members of the Church of England.

As I noted in chapter 4, this is an example of what Reverends Emily Swan and Ken Wilson were referring to in their book *Solus Jesus*, when they stated that over the past five hundred years, White, male, educated men of power interpreted Scripture.[29] The same is true, for the most part, today. So again, we can't be afraid to question what we are taught to believe when it feels wrong.

I know with certainty that regardless of his marital status, there is no way Jesus would condone or be complicit with the mistreatment, subjugation, or abuse of women and girls or men and boys. These self-obsessed, hurtful, and demeaning behaviors are not aligned with loving one another as Jesus wants us to. Therefore, I believe Jesus would want both women and men to focus on the spiritual and social obligations we have to be responsible for ourselves, so that we treat other people as we want to be treated.

9

We Need to Talk about Sex

One day, when I was living in Birmingham, Alabama, I was edging the lawn of the house I rented. With string trimmer in hand, I moved to the side yard and began working on the little strip of grass between the sidewalk and street. For some reason I looked up and was stunned to see a man in a house across the street standing behind his screen door. He was completely naked and clearly masturbating in full view of anyone passing by; in fact, given the way he was standing in a fully lit doorway with nothing but a screen in front of him, he seemed to be making a show of it, as if he wanted to make sure we saw him.

I was too traumatized to say anything to the man in the moment. But later my three housemates and I confronted him about his behavior, and the man moved soon afterward.

The audacity of forcing someone to be an unwilling participant in our sexual behavior—be it something as relatively minor as what this man did or as major as physical sexual assault—must not go unchecked. We need to get to the root of the problem as to why our male-dominated society tolerates so much unacceptable sexual conduct and aggression.

The #MeToo movement that began online in 2006 exposed the vast world of male sexual misbehavior by shining a spotlight

We Need to Talk about Sex

on men in all walks of life, from leaders of companies to pizza parlor managers, from entertainment icons to church officials and politicians. Following the woman-affirming example of Jesus, Christians should be the first to speak out against people forcing themselves upon *anyone*. We must actively demand men and boys accept sexual responsibility not only for themselves but also for family members, coworkers, fellow church members, partners, sports teammates, business leaders, politicians, and friends.

We must set a positive example and challenge everyone who thinks it is acceptable to call any woman a "slut," "prude," "bitch," "jezebel," or any other insulting name. Or to make jokes about women being "barefoot and pregnant." Or to tell women to get back in the kitchen. Or to make derogatory remarks about women drivers. Let's join forces and oppose the actions of men who talk over or interrupt women, or offer unwelcome comments about women's bodies, or manspread (sitting crotch out with legs spread wide in a way that intrudes on the space of others).

In a world in which men and boys are not held accountable, a woman or girl who speaks out against sexual abuses of power is often intimidated into remaining silent about abuses, threatened with more physical harm, or blamed for the assault. When star high school and college male athletes as well as professionals are found guilty of rape, their families plead for leniency because they "have a bright future." What about the future of the women they violate who have the courage to speak out?

I was eleven when a sixteen-year-old male babysitter sexually molested me. When I begged him to stop, he threatened, "I'll cut your tits off if you ever tell anyone what I am doing."

In high school, while on a church hayride, a teenage boy wanted to molest me under a blanket. I told him no. He said his father had instructed him to try with every girl until he found one who would do as he wanted. I did not tell anyone.

CHAPTER 9

You know from chapter 4 I was eighteen when a physician casually ordered his nurse to leave the room so he would be free to sexually molest me in private. When I came forward about what the physician did, I was dismissed as just one more in a very long line of women and teenage girls he routinely abused; that was "just the way he was."

In my early twenties, I was walking with a friend when a man leaned out of his truck window and screamed, "Hey lesbos! All you need is a good FUCK to straighten you out." It was just one of many similar verbal assaults hurled at me.

As a grown woman, I was threatened with the termination of my job at a Christian college if I exposed the sexual misconduct of one of the bosses, who was accused of assaulting a fellow employee and several female students. Male college administrators refused to address the accusations. It was well known among students and staff that several of these men were guilty of the same inexcusable behavior. Female administrators feared losing their jobs should they speak up.

As a mature woman, I occasionally receive unsolicited messages from men who send photos of their genitals, videos of them masturbating, and crude sexual references designed to remind me of my "place" as something that exists to amuse them, gratify them, or make them feel powerful.

Sex, like religion, should never be used as a weapon against anyone—especially within the church. But sadly, we all know exploitation is rampant in religious circles.

In 2003, the *Boston Globe* won a Pulitzer Prize for its series (which would eventually grow to over eight hundred articles) that brought the sexual abuse of hundreds of children by Catholic priests—and the decades-long cover-up—into the national spotlight.[30] The widespread abuse of boys and girls alike soon became an international story with victims speaking up across the world.

A 2021 third-party investigation of the Southern Baptist Convention revealed that leadership buried multiple sex-abuse claims for more than twenty years. They ignored accusations and slandered and intimidated sex-abuse survivors to protect the church from legal liability. Over 380 pastors affiliated with the Southern Baptist Convention were accused of sexual abuse.[31]

Russell D. Moore, an American theologian, ethicist, and preacher, reacted to the news:

> I was wrong to call sexual abuse in the Southern Baptist Convention . . . a crisis. *Crisis* is too small a word. It is an apocalypse. . . .
>
> The investigation uncovers a reality far more evil and systematic than I imagined it could be. . . .
>
> I only know firsthand the rage of one who wonders while reading what happened on the seventh floor of that Southern Baptist building, how many children were raped, how many people were assaulted, how many screams were silenced, while we boasted that no one could reach the world for Jesus like we could.
>
> That's more than a crisis. It's even more than just a crime. It's blasphemy. And anyone who cares about heaven ought to be mad as hell.[32]

It adversely affects society when any man or woman denies, without seeking and considering credible evidence, the validity of claims of any victim who courageously comes forward to report sexual abuse.

It adversely affects society when the double standard of "he's a stud, she's a slut" reigns supreme and men and boys are expected

CHAPTER 9

to be the initiators of sexual activity while women and girls are expected to remain pure and untouched until marriage.

It adversely affects society when many men and boys are so insecure and confused about what it means to be a man that they attempt to build themselves up through domination, aggression, and sexual abuse because they've been taught this is what it means to be male.

Wouldn't Jesus evaluate this as one of the huge failures of Christianity, the church, and human society in general?

You might be thinking, "The church does a good job of shaming people for sexual behavior already," and you'd be right, but that leads to my second point: There is an obvious and important difference between consensual and nonconsensual acts. We must be willing to fight against one without denigrating the other.

Let's start with the taboo of masturbation. The fact is, sex feels good to most people. Our bodies were designed this way. People who responsibly pleasure themselves, without taking advantage of, forcing themselves on, or hurting anyone, are not going to hell. We don't end up blind. Our sex organs don't fall off. Our relationship to God does not break or become diminished. In fact, with overwhelming numbers of sexual abuse allegations in the Catholic Church against members of the clergy, who must take a vow of celibacy, it seems there is a solid case for encouraging a little *more* sexual self-love.

God designed us to feel our way through life. Nothing positive comes from attempting to deny our natural feelings. But being respectful of our bodies and respecting the rights of others over their bodies are cornerstones of a healthy society.

And this respect of the rights of others over their own bodies extends to health care as well.

I happen to believe that Jesus, who considered women his equals, would confront our male-dominated church, government, and society about why there is an effort to maintain control over women and their right to make reproductive decisions over their bodies.

Let me be clear: *I, Regina Victoria Cates, am not a promoter of abortion.*

I think abortion is a terrible, heart-wrenching decision for everyone involved, and I would never treat it as something trivial or convenient.

I am, however, a firm believer in an individual's control over their own body. I am an advocate of women's reproductive rights, including a woman's decision to end a pregnancy. I support birth control and sex education as crucial for a healthy society. I am an ardent proponent of women preventing unplanned pregnancy. I support men being sexually responsible, including wearing condoms and having vasectomies. It is precisely *because of my faith* that I see it as vital for the Christian church to focus on sexual responsibility to prevent unplanned pregnancy—not only as a spiritual necessity but also as a logical and loving social responsibility, to ensure a healthy population balance for the earth and the best care of all children.

And I am confident Jesus would not want me, or anyone, to sit in judgment over, or to attempt to control, the reproductive health options women choose for themselves.

You may remember my friend Tim, a retired Christian minister. I reached out to him for his thoughts on this question. His assessment? Based on everything we know from the Gospels, Jesus would support compassion and understanding rather than suppression of a woman's right to make her own decisions. Tim writes (in an email to me on July 22, 2019):

> As a young minister, I learned early on not every moral issue is black and white. There is so much gray that covers the

CHAPTER 9

choices we make in life. I'm convinced most people who are so aggressively opposed to abortion have never been confronted with an unwanted pregnancy, a tragic medical and sometimes fatal defect identified in a fetus, or an expectant mother with a life-threatening disease.

I have. And these are excruciating experiences for all involved, especially the mother.

In more than twenty years as a minister serving four congregations, I found myself with families facing horrible choices regarding a woman's pregnancy. For those who chose to end it, I felt nothing but compassion, hurt, and sorrow for them. Never once did any of the girls or women I dealt with facing an abortion ever take it lightly. They did not breeze casually through it, or think it insignificant. They all suffered through the decision, yet each determined it was what was best for them and their pregnancy.

In my heart, I believe Jesus would hold a woman's hand in this situation and grieve with her. There would be no shaming, no judgment, no withdrawing of affection or love. That is what I see in his teaching and in the way he lived.

Christians must stop describing Jesus in terms of political power, sanctimonious blather, raw prejudice, and cruel condemnation. These are not the characteristics of the Jesus of scripture and history who demonstrated unconditional acceptance of people in the worst circumstances imaginable.

Let the crucifixion guide us in these complex matters. There Jesus died unjustly, brutally, miserably, and yet, he died generously, with a clear open heart. His death said, even if you kill me, I will still love you.

That is transcendent love. A love that goes beyond moral rules, beyond Church precepts, beyond political expediency, beyond all boundaries.

We Need to Talk about Sex

The love being written about here. It frees the oppressed. It unburdens the guilty. It honors women. It personifies equality. It says if you will love like this, all people will be sacred to you.

The church has the duty to lead us to treat one another with Jesus-like love and compassion. This requires all of us to honestly question our role, and that of the church, in defending or participating in dictatorial behavior, no matter our personal beliefs. Christianity as a whole must vilify the behavior of any group of misguided people who use violence in the name of God. Demanding people believe as we do, shouting verbal abuse at women walking into clinics, bombing women's clinics, murdering their doctors and staff, setting fire to their buildings—these are actions designed to terrorize people. I believe Jesus would be bewildered and enraged that any Christian could possibly believe God would be part of any terrorist organization anywhere. Not everyone is as radical or extreme as some anti-abortion groups, but I firmly believe Jesus would remind all of us that terrorists and dictators are not doing God's work. *Ever.*

In addition, the church must be proactive by providing ample opportunity for women and men alike to prevent pregnancy by confronting its lack of support for funding sex-education programs that teach sexual responsibility and respect for one another.

The church must also face the patriarchal hypocrisy of demanding women give birth while ignoring any responsibility the church has to love, educate, and feed the children they are forcing to be born. Forced birth is not pro-life. In the words of Benedictine nun Sister Joan Chittister:

> I don't believe that just because you're opposed to abortion that makes you pro-life. In fact, I think in many cases, your

CHAPTER 9

morality is deeply lacking if all you want is a child born but not a child fed, not a child educated, not a child housed. And why would I think that you aren't pro-life? Because you don't want any tax money to go there. That's not pro-life. That's pro-birth. We need a much broader conversation on what the morality of pro-life is.[33]

Wouldn't Jesus want us to admit the conversation needs to be much bigger than we've made it?

Pastor Dave Barnhart, of Saint Junia United Methodist Church in Birmingham, Alabama, passionately believes Jesus would view the issue in far more complex and nuanced ways. His thoughts (originally shared on Facebook on June 25, 2018) went viral on social media in May 2022.

> The unborn are a convenient group of people to advocate for.
>
> They never make demands of you; they are morally uncomplicated, unlike the incarcerated, addicted, or the chronically poor; they don't resent your condescension or complain that you are not politically correct; unlike widows, they don't ask you to question patriarchy; unlike orphans, they don't need money, education, or childcare; unlike aliens, they don't bring all that racial, cultural, and religious baggage that you dislike; they allow you to feel good about yourself without any work at creating or maintaining relationships; and when they are born, you can forget about them, because they cease to be unborn.
>
> It's almost as if, by being born, they have died to you. You can love the unborn and advocate for them without substantially challenging your own wealth, power, or privilege, without re-imagining social structures, apologizing, or making reparations to anyone.

We Need to Talk about Sex

They are, in short, the perfect people to love if you want to claim to love Jesus but actually dislike people who breathe. Prisoners? Immigrants? The sick? The poor? Widows? Orphans? All the groups that are specifically mentioned in the Bible? They all get thrown under the bus for the unborn.

Whether we want to admit it or not, abortion is not uncommon in the church; women just don't want to talk about it. A 2015 study conducted by Care Net and Lifeway Research was quite extensive, with approximately ninety questions answered by 1,038 women from across the country. According to the study, 70 percent of women (seven in ten) who have had an abortion indicate their religious preference as Christian. Fifty-two percent of churchgoers who have had an abortion say no one at church knows they terminated a pregnancy.[34]

We also need to realize there is much misinformation and many myths about abortion, such as that every woman who obtains an abortion later regrets it. A large, long-term study called the Turnaway Study tracked the mental health of nearly one thousand women in twenty-one states who wanted and received an abortion between 2008 and 2010.[35] The women were interviewed every six months over the next five years. At the end of that time, 99 percent of the women who had an abortion believed they had made the right decision—in fact, relief was the prominent emotion.

The Turnaway Study also looked at the impacts of being denied an abortion. Results showed women who were turned away were more likely to experience significant anxiety and stress. Social psychologist Antonia Biggs, one of the Turnaway researchers from the Advancing New Standards in Reproductive Health project at the University of California, San Francisco, notes, "In

CHAPTER 9

my research what we found is that the challenges of getting an abortion—finding a place, traveling, having to disclose your abortion to someone you would have preferred not to—increased symptoms of depression, anxiety and stress."[36]

In addition to admitting the hypocrisy and misinformation surrounding abortion, we also need to acknowledge that attempts to limit the rights of women over their bodies and reproductive choices continue to perpetuate an ancient patriarchal fear, one that is summed up by Leonard Shlain: "Millennia ago males intentionally set themselves above females when they realized women were the only ones capable of birthing new life. Today we continue to live under patriarchal societies with sets of institutionalized social rules put in place by men to control the sexual and reproductive rights of women."[37]

Reverend Britt Skarda, retired senior pastor of Pulaski Heights United Methodist Church in Little Rock, Arkansas, believes fear, domination, and control were never rational or spiritually acceptable excuses to God or Jesus for males to create and perpetuate a misogynistic rule over women and girls. That rule includes continued efforts to control female reproductive choices.

Skarda says in a February 13, 2023, email:

> The effects of patriarchy in the early church can be seen in practices that favored the rights of fathers to prevent abortion over the rights of mothers to make decisions related to their reproductive health. This was especially true in the Roman Empire. Essentially, laws and practices in the early Christian Church were more concerned with a father's desire for an heir than the needs of the mother or the fetus. Even now these decisions are being determined by male-dominated institutions.

We Need to Talk about Sex

In the United States today, matters related to abortion are driven less by biblical scholarship and theological understanding and more by partisan politics. Fifty years ago, both political parties were pretty much on the same page with regard to abortion. Democrats and Republicans approved or disapproved of abortion at about the same rate. In 1969, ninety percent of all Baptists in the state of Texas approved of abortion at some stage in a pregnancy. The shift came with the 1972 presidential campaign of Richard M. Nixon. Nixon decided to take an anti-abortion position as a way of appealing to Catholic voters, as well as other social conservatives.

The Republican Party took up abortion as a way of arguing that they were the party of God that truly cared about life from conception. This move was intended to brand the Republican party as pro-family. As a result, extremist factions within the Republican party today have not only overturned Roe v. Wade, they desire to prevent a woman from having an abortion in the case of rape or incest, as well as situations where the woman's life is in danger.

Jesus, on the other hand, would proclaim that life, in all of its beauty and ugliness, is not a black or white matter. Rather, life is crammed full of gray areas in which life conflicts with life. Jesus would welcome and embrace the freedom of a woman to make life-changing decisions regarding her body and her health.

As far as "pro-life" Christians who believe that life begins with the fetus, yet seem to care little for the life/health/wellbeing of the woman/girl carrying the child, it honestly has little to do with faith. It's all about politics.

What would Jesus say about these people? Maybe something like this:

CHAPTER 9

"How can you love a fetus you cannot see when you fail to love the woman you can see who is carrying that fetus?"

It takes a single focus to end a double standard. To cultivate women and men who view themselves as equal children of God requires acknowledging that God's plan for human beings was not domination or control but harmony, with men and women living in partnership rather than hierarchy. We need to define masculinity not as a force that conquers but as one that empowers.

My friend Charles labors to walk in the footsteps of Jesus, so when I asked what he believes it means to be a man and how men are to treat women, his response in a June 15, 2019, email was very much in line with what I believe Jesus taught:

> A friend of mine once pointed out that in the movie scenes of my life, I'm in every scene and of course I'm going to think life is about me and how I feel. If I think everything is about me and my feelings, I will project this self-focus into how I act as a man and how I treat others. I will get angry because I didn't get what I wanted and someone owes me more respect than I was shown. I will get jealous because someone got something that I didn't. I become greedy because what I have is mine and all mine. I feel guilty because I didn't do what I thought I should and now I owe someone something. Attitudes of anger, jealousy, greed, and guilt are all reflections of how I see myself in light of others around me. My experience and observation is that this is not healthy, for myself or others.
>
> The #MeToo movement recognizes and fights against the unhealthy outcome of this self-focused attitude. Said an-

other way and to paraphrase an ancient book, "don't merely look out for your own personal interest but also the interests of others." Simple to say, hard to do. With this in mind, I start with a definition that I don't claim as my own.

I embrace a definition for manhood that incorporates efforts to live out four characteristics in light of life not being just about me: 1) Reject passivity; 2) Accept responsibility; 3) Lead courageously; 4) Invest eternally. By injecting these qualities into the everyday decision-making process, the resulting actions reflect what it means to me to be a man.

So how does this play out in how a man treats women? Incorporate these same concepts. Reject passivity, accept responsibility, lead courageously, and invest eternally, into the relationship. It's a relationship, don't miss this. Consider her interests as well as yours. Ask questions. Listen to the answers. Protect the relationship. Act honorably. Give freely. Encourage. Serve one another. Accept one another. Be patient. Be hospitable. Care.

Simple, but not easy.

Contrary to what many talking heads in the media would have you believe, supporting women does not mean suppressing men. It means we instill within our men and boys a vision of inner strength that emphasizes honesty, respect, and responsibility. We impart self-confidence and humility in men and boys rather than encourage the wounded ego's self-focus of dominance and arrogance.

This is what another friend, David, believes is the solution to end what he views as universal toxic masculinity. In his words to me by email on May 29, 2019:

CHAPTER 9

As a society we must have the courage to question the bill of goods we've been sold about what is manly. It's absolutely incumbent on us to challenge all of the established beliefs about the traditional toxic masculinity of the macho, he-man, tough-guy image. We must try with all sincerity to understand the fear-based mindset from which those beliefs came.

So, men: let's not underestimate the power of the feminine but welcome it into our lives. Let's treat women with the utmost respect and honor and seek their help in all things, because without them we can only ever be half as good as we really could be.

With the emergence of the #MeToo movement it's clear we are now, once and for all, on notice. The "boys will be boys" behavioral narrative will no longer be an acceptable excuse for our inexcusable behavior, and rightfully so.

I often wonder whether modern-day preachers would tell Jesus to "take it like a man" when he was betrayed, ridiculed, scapegoated, and abandoned by those who professed to love him. Or when he was beaten with the cat-o'-nine-tails whip. Or when he repeatedly fell while being forced to carry the heavy wooden cross of his execution. Or when he was nailed to the cross to hang until dead. He didn't fight back, but he wasn't emotionless, either.

We know Jesus was capable of deep feelings and emotion. He cried over people who rejected God's peace (Luke 19:41). He wept at the death of a dear friend (John 11:35). He suffered deep anguish and sorrow at the thought of his impending death (Matthew 26; Luke 22). He cried out in agony on the cross (Matthew 27:46; Mark 15:34).

I don't believe anyone would call Jesus a "momma's boy" or a wimp. And yet, somehow, we've shamed men and boys for ex-

We Need to Talk about Sex

pressing any emotion but anger. How does the cruel practice of teaching boys to "take it like a man" help fashion men who are caring and gentle, let alone self-confident and well adjusted?

I have wondered:

Does circumcision negatively impact our boys and men?

Does it leave some consciously or unconsciously angry that they had no choice over their own body?

I don't know the answers, but as someone whose body holds memories of traumatic physical injury and abuse, I wonder. Maybe it is time for us to collectively ask ourselves these hard questions since circumcision is not laid down as a requirement in the New Testament. Instead, Christians are urged, "When you came to Christ, you were 'circumcised,' but not by a physical procedure. Christ performed a spiritual circumcision—the cutting away of your sinful nature" (Colossians 2:11–12 NLT).

We will not advance our collective human potential or grow our spiritual awareness by continuing down the same macho, he-man path of our ancestors—even if those ancestors are our parents or grandparents. To end sexism, misogyny, and sexual abuse we must address our part in creating and supporting a culture where sex is power.

My friend Chris is someone Jesus would be proud to call friend. As a loving husband and gentle father of a daughter and son, he is a hands-on proponent of gender equity and ending the image of women being viewed as sexual objects. He is a Christian, and his faith has led him to believe he needs to continually check his own behaviors and beliefs. In an email to me on May 28, 2019, he wrote,

> I am a big sports fan and I often listen to a popular sports talk-show host, Colin Cowherd. Cowherd often uses this say-

CHAPTER 9

ing, "I don't want to be right, I want to get it right." So often male sports fans state their opinion and look for any piece of evidence to support them being right, while ignoring any evidence to the contrary. The smart male fan is the one who is willing to say he was wrong and to change his opinion to get it right.

We should extend this mantra beyond sports to all walks of life, especially to one of the most important social issues we face, which has been brought to light by the #MeToo movement. Women are often objectified and this has resulted in an abundance of sexual harassment and sexual assault. Unfortunately, society has perpetuated this objectification. For example, women are portrayed as sex symbols in movies, social media influencers are using provocative photos to sell more products, and who can ignore the impact of the pornography industry? I don't pretend I am impervious to the effects of these influences on my own views of women. But, this is where the willingness of a man to listen and change becomes so important.

Are we as men willing to listen to facts that are contradictory to what we want to believe, accept them, and adjust our perspective accordingly? Are we willing to get it right or do we just want to be right? If we want to truly be men, if we want to get it right, then we need to be open to hearing the stories of women who have been mistreated and we need to change how we act and treat women to avoid making the same mistakes again.

To create lasting equity, we must first awaken to the reality in which we live. To love Jesus and love one another as Jesus asks, it makes sense for the church to play a key role in fostering an appreciation of this responsibility. Let's release ourselves from patriarchy and misogyny by owning up to them. Let's care that Jesus would ask what we did within our hearts, families, churches, communities, and governments to end the sexual, financial, and psychological abuse and domination of women and girls.

The church can help build lasting gender equity by refusing to label God as exclusively male. The church can change the future by ensuring it does not repeat the mistakes of the past by covering up, ignoring, or perpetuating sexual abuse. The church can lead the way in teaching what it means to be emotionally healthy men and women alike. But the church has to be willing to live like Jesus first.

10

Superheroes Are Real

Superheroes are not only the subjects of fantastical stories or the daydreams of sad little girls trapped in fundamentalism; they can also be normal people. In fact, we are surrounded by them; they simply look different from how we may imagine. They don't wear capes, have X-ray vision, or shoot lightning bolts from their fingers. They look like you and me and our next-door neighbors. Real-life superheroes use their powers of integrity, insight, and inclusiveness to help the world become a better place. And some of our most influential superheroes are those who dedicate themselves to servant leadership in government.

I was thirteen when my father took me on a day trip to Austin to tour the state capital. One of our stops was the Texas Senate, the upper house of the state legislature. The official proceedings captured my attention, as did one senator in particular, Barbara Jordan. She was the first Black woman elected to the Texas Senate. Her record was one of public service with authenticity, empathy, and courage.

Maybe Dad hoped the experience would ignite a desire within me to someday run for office. Growing up, I remember my parents actively supporting the women and men alike who they believed were best qualified to fill leadership positions in local, state, and national government. While I did not pursue a career in government, my parents' enthusiasm did help cultivate within me a deep appreciation for the honesty and dedication of sincere public servants who work to uphold justice for all citizens and promote the common welfare of all.

Regardless of political party affiliation, true public servants—people who serve the public—have a verifiable record of accomplishments that have bettered the lives of the public they serve. They are required either to swear on a religious book or to affirm a nonreligious oath of office, which legally binds them to protect our right to liberty and the pursuit of happiness. They are bound to defend our freedom from unjust laws, rigged and discriminatory voting systems, and a tyrannical government. They have a duty to keep church and state separate, to safeguard us against those who twist their distorted religious ideas of an omnipotent being to press agendas of inequality, control, and prejudice.

Leaders of integrity are those who encourage principled excellence among their colleagues and constituents. They consistently behave in ways that reflect the values of honorable character. They apply the same standards of behavior to their own political party that they do to those they view as opponents. True servant leaders know that for a system of democracy to work, our governmental representatives have to be diverse. Genuine public servants, whether Democrat, Independent, or Republican, are willing to cross the aisle to do what is best for the country and its variety of citizens. They share power and use the political influence they have on behalf of those who most need their help. And they guard against anyone, themselves included, who abuses positions of power.

Regardless of an individual's religious beliefs, a true public servant is a model of Christlike living because Jesus was a public

CHAPTER 10

servant. Even though he did not serve in government, Jesus is considered one of the most famous servant leaders in history who devoted, and gave, his life to better the lives of people. While I would never propose that we impose that comparison on someone who is not Christian, those of us who do strive to follow Jesus can look to leaders of deep integrity as modern-day examples of his philosophies of servant leadership.

Christ modeled unity, support, and honor. He treasured justice, discernment, and forethought. He acted with humility, charity, and accountability. Trustworthiness, inclusivity, and self-discipline were important behaviors to him. However, Jesus was not a politician. He was not motivated by fame, fortune, or power. He did not promote himself. Jesus did not serve humanity with the goal of having a religion created for him. Rather, his desire was to aid people from a place of respect and empathy, which he consistently displayed through the decency of his character. Operating from truthfulness, compassion, and honor made Christ a great leader and an enduring inspiration.

I believe Jesus would question why we don't value honorable character as our most important characteristic in today's political climate and as the most significant aspect of those we select for leadership positions. We need to ask ourselves some tough questions about what being a great leader would mean to Jesus and what great leadership should mean to us as his admirers. It seems many of us who claim to love Jesus have forgotten, or never knew, the spiritual responsibility we have to God to be people of honor, peace, and empathy and the obligation we have to God to fashion a world guided by governmental leaders who inspire us to be honest, responsible, and inclusive, too.

Do we believe Jesus would disregard ethics and relevant experience in considering what makes one qualified for a leadership position?

Superheroes Are Real

The study of effective leadership is my specialty. I hold a master's degree in the subject, having spent three years studying public and private management in graduate school, on top of several decades spent running both for-profit and not-for-profit organizations. I was privileged to manage, recruit, and train staff and allocate budgets. I wrote and implemented long-term strategic and marketing plans. As a leader, I was the face of the organization and served as liaison to other organizations. While I readily admit I don't know everything, through my years of experience, I have learned a few key points about what does and does not work in leadership.

Effective leaders know that without open and honest communication, no trust will be built. Without trust, there will be no success for the leadership.

Organizations, whether in business or government, don't succeed long-term if the goals of the leaders differ from the goals of the majority of shareholders—or the majority of citizens in our representative democracy.

Listening to people, from the lowest to highest levels of the organization, is mandatory for decision makers. Without awareness of and caring about the needs of the people who make up an organization (or the majority of citizens), no leadership will be effective or last any length of time.

But the most important lesson I have learned in selecting effective and trustworthy leaders is recognizing that ethical, moral, and legal integrity begins at the top. Leaders of integrity raise the personal conduct of those within the organization. They are fair and honest, have empathy for people, and are skilled at conflict resolution and peacekeeping. Trustworthy leaders enhance the credibility of the organization within the minds of those they serve and remain people of honorable character.

CHAPTER 10

No matter what position of authority someone holds, to be great, she or he has to be committed to honesty, respect, and responsibility. In order to love Jesus, who was the gold standard of leading with integrity, our spiritual obligation is to align our behavior with the values of integrity, too.

Of course, we are not going to be perfect. Neither will our leaders. However, Christ would remind us, in order to be a great nation and world, we have to be governed by women and men of great integrity. This means *we cannot make Jesus-like, principled decisions about someone's integrity based solely on the fact that they belong to the political party we side with*. Jesus wants us to do our homework and recognize genuine public servants, those who have a verifiable record of honest and just service to the majority of citizens. When no candidate within our own political party offers true integrity, we look beyond party affiliation to vote for someone who listens and is committed to trustworthiness, reverence, and accountability.

Jesus was killed by those who did not value different points of view, religious beliefs, or living with integrity. They did not value social justice. Those in political and religious power viewed Christ's honorable-servant approach to leadership as a threat to the authoritarian grasp they held over the masses. The rulers were intimidated because Jesus valued leaders who served and protected the human rights of the people. No matter if it was government, religion, or challenging social norms, Jesus was not shy about calling out those who abused their positions of power over people.

Jesus made it clear that the autocratic desire of his apostles to rule was unacceptable. His need was for them to be thoughtful servant leaders. To fashion an effective representative democracy, we have the same need. We have to be governed by women and men of principle who are brave and bold yet humble. They are respectful of the connection they have with those they lead. Women and men of integrity *want* to be held accountable for the influence they have over us.

Therefore, Jesus would not believe those who work to limit people's human rights or sow divisiveness and chaos are great leaders. He would not set people up to lose so he could win. An honorable person, Jesus did not lie, cheat, or use his position for his own gain. He did not abuse people. Jesus would not deny science and fact. He would not label factual news fake. He would not cut other people down in an attempt to raise himself up. And Jesus would not place value in or trust people who spread misinformation, disinformation, false equivalencies, and conspiracy theories or promote bullying, corruption, division, and violence.

During one election cycle, a man came to my door campaigning for a local politician who was running for state office. The man spoke for a few minutes about the candidate's qualifications and handed me a flyer. He asked if his candidate had my vote. I told him I wanted to investigate the candidate further, to do my own research, in order to make the most informed decision. Faced with my noncommittal response, the man began to badmouth his candidate's opponent. I politely and firmly told the man canvasing for the candidate, "I believe the most important work we undertake, whether it is in politics or everyday life, is to learn to deal with our differing views by behaving in courteous and fact-based ways, rather than tearing one another down."

What kind of shallow, irresponsible, and uninformed people would we be if we allowed ourselves to be influenced by someone who tears down an opponent or opposing political party?

Wouldn't Jesus demand better from us?

CHAPTER 10

We must learn to differentiate between constructive critique (logical, fact-based, and respectful) and opinion, lies, and divisive trash talk aimed at destroying other people in an effort to build up a political party or a candidate's ego or to feed a public figure who trash-talks because they are addicted to the attention and illusion of power their conduct brings.

To be right with Jesus, we need to care to be informed. In order to make decisions based on what Jesus would do, we need to be knowledgeable of the facts about the issues and the people we entrust with leadership positions, whether in government or elsewhere. To do so, we must discern: who is serving our democracy, and who is undermining it?

One of my first jobs after college was as director of classified advertising for the *Columbia Missourian* newspaper. Part of my responsibility was to supervise journalism students who were enrolled in the University of Missouri School of Journalism. In order to be well rounded, they were required to work in different divisions of the newspaper, including advertising. Upon graduation, some of these young people wanted to pursue careers as investigative journalists. They chose reporting because they wanted to make the world a better place by helping expose corruption, greed, dishonesty, and phony news and to report on matters of interest and safety to the public.

Through the experience of working with journalism professionals and students, I came to admire the depth of due diligence and honor required to be an investigative journalist with integrity. These people were not tabloid ambulance chasers. They were not vendors of fake news, conspiracy theories, or half-truths. They did not spread gossip, lie intentionally, or vilify people. They did not deliberately mislead people because of some hidden agenda or for money. They worked hard to avoid confirmation bias. They were not erratic, lazy, or prejudiced in their reporting. They dug deep to uncover tangible facts, to cite multiple sources, to ensure what they reported was true and verifiable.

It is because of women and men who are seasoned fact-finding reporters that you and I have access to the truth. Each day countless people of honor work hard to ensure truth speaks to power. To alert us to evil people doing evil things. To get the facts straight. To present us with information so we can be informed about matters that concern all of us.

Shouldn't we care to be informed of the truth and reality?

There is no such thing as "alternative facts." Facts don't change because someone misrepresents or misconstrues evidence or misuses books like the Bible to support their position or views. Jesus would be disappointed by those who say they love him but who are deaf to this slanderous and fraudulent irresponsibility. Jesus would remind us gossip, bullying, and tearing people down are never aligned with what he taught. He would question why anyone would allow themselves to be influenced by opinionated news, anti-science theories, and false political attack ads designed to defame people. Lying, falsifying information, and denying access to information are tools of oppression and tyranny.

He would clearly state that the practice of misrepresenting an opponent's position is "bearing false witness." We need to heed the wisdom of US District Judge Amy Berman Jackson, who said, "Politics don't corrupt people. People corrupt politics."[38]

Sowing division, chaos, and misinformation is not the behavior of great leaders or people of integrity. Nothing positive is added to our democratic process when we reward our representatives (or *their* representatives) for slandering opponents. Name calling and attack ads are cheap political tricks. Mistaking opinionated commentary for truth only results in our being

CHAPTER 10

uninformed to the facts. Allowing ourselves to be manipulated by salacious, clickbait, facts-optional claims about candidates, or people in general, is admitting we are not interested in thoughtful investigation that may go against our pre-existing biases, and that means we are not interested in truth.

Historian and professor Heather Cox-Richardson discusses the 2023 derailment of Norfolk Southern train cars and subsequent release of toxic chemicals near East Palestine, Ohio, near the Ohio-Pennsylvania border, as one example of how we are being lied to and kept in the dark when the bottom line of a large corporation or the big-government agenda of bought-and-paid-for politicians is threatened.

> Pennsylvania governor Josh Shapiro, a Democrat, said that Norfolk Southern had botched its response to the accident. "Norfolk Southern has repeatedly assured us of the safety of their rail cars—in fact, leading Norfolk Southern personnel described them to me as 'the Cadillac of rail cars'—yet despite these assertions, these were the same cars that Norfolk Southern personnel rushed to vent and burn without gathering input from state and local leaders. Norfolk Southern's well-known opposition to modern regulations [requires] further scrutiny and investigation to limit the devastating effects of future accidents on people's lives, property, businesses, and the environment."
>
> Shapiro was likely referring to the fact that in 2017, after donors from the railroad industry poured more than $6 million into Republican political campaigns, the Trump administration got rid of a rule imposed by the Obama administration that required better braking systems on rail cars that carried hazardous flammable materials.[39]

Superheroes Are Real

This one incident, out of thousands, illustrates the need for us to care when we are systematically being "played" by those who bow to and protect the interests of their big-dollar donors. Countless disinformation narratives are created by paid-for elected officials who don't actually govern for the "people" but for their own special interests.

But when the truth of their actions is revealed, they deny, spin, create a counternarrative or false narrative, and go on the attack.

Jesus did not lie, slander, exaggerate, or place blame elsewhere. He would not find dishonesty and tearing people down in an attempt to build ourselves up suitable or benign behavior. Jesus would not consider anyone who bad-mouths people or who does not take responsibility for the health and safety of all people to be leadership material. He would not be okay with anyone betraying their integrity in favor of a cult leader who spreads division and praises dishonor. This type of bullying is never moral, ethical, or acceptable to God, to Jesus, or to a healthy society. If we don't care about truth and respect, aren't we crucifying the very values of integrity (respect, honesty, cooperation, etc.) that Jesus held dear?

As citizens, we hold much responsibility for the way intimidation and the vilification of those perceived to be opponents have become so widespread. By not raising a unified voice to decry these practices within our sphere of influence, we have allowed negativity and denigration of others to seep into every part of life. The epidemic of disrespect throughout our political, social, and entertainment environments would be embarrassing to Jesus. It is never Christlike to attack those we have disagreements with or who are different from us. We cannot love Jesus and sit by, ignoring the real potential our silence has to perpetuate this damaging behavior.

CHAPTER 10

Although we may live in a free country and have freedom of speech, we are not entitled to say what we want without regard to the consequences of our actions, whether in spoken conversation, text, print, social-media post, or on television. Actions without forethought and accountability are not free. There are always consequences, as our God-given gift of free will comes with a great amount of personal responsibility. Only by being accountable for our actions do we maintain our integrity as we navigate social systems that often allow and encourage pushing acceptable boundaries to intolerable, ridiculous, and dangerous extremes. There is an old expression that states, "My rights end where yours begin." With this in mind, we must acknowledge that hate speech is not free speech when it encourages behavior and policies that harm other people.

Don't personal freedom and God's gift of free will require us to operate at the highest levels of responsibility?

Don't we need to admit that vast billion-dollar social media companies fuel anger, division, chaos, and violence?

"Treat people as we want to be treated" clearly means we are charged by God with creating a world where we, our children, our neighbors, and our public servants are safe from being bullied, lied about, and derided. We can create the safe and respectful attitude God wants us to extend to one another by acknowledging the egotistical motivation behind all trash talk. No matter on what platform divisive speech is delivered, or by whom, we turn this wickedness off. We refuse to attend such rallies or church services. We walk away when someone starts spewing this abuse. When those who lie and vilify others lose their audience, they lose their influence. However, we have to work together to achieve this goal.

God is asking each of us to actively bring about this positive change. We can absolutely be superheroes. Being a citizen of a representative democracy comes with great responsibility.

Superheroes Are Real

God gave us a huge gift in our ability to think critically, not in a negative or condescending way, but with the power to objectively evaluate, through the integrity and logic of soul, whom and what we see, read, or hear. From the moment a person steps onto the political scene, we—the citizens who have the power to put them in office or remove them from it—are charged with making certain, through our own due diligence, that a candidate's words and actions are truthful. We are to look fairly and listen carefully. We accept that these women and men will not be perfect, but they will admit their mistakes and commit to doing better.

As we fill every position of responsibility, our job is to seek credible information about the candidate's record of behavior, upon which we can base a "what Jesus would do" decision about them or one of their political appointees. The integrity of our souls is not biased along political party lines or positions of leadership responsibility. Integrity of soul is focused only on making certain someone we support is worthy of the backing of Jesus, too. We cannot allow ourselves to make excuses for unethical and irresponsible people, no matter how they promise to make our lives better, safer, or richer. Our lives shouldn't feel easier or more fulfilling when people suffer injustice and inequity.

Integrity-driven people who truly love and honor Jesus don't use the Bible to weave a "divine vessel" theology around a political candidate, and certainly not around anyone whose history is void of the honorable character of Jesus.

God gave us power over the choices we make. That means God is not in control of our country or world politics. If God were in control, people of honorable integrity would be serving in governments around the world. Peace and love would rain down. Therefore, we the people are charged by God to recognize and support true leaders of integrity, Christian and non-Christian alike.

To honor Jesus, we must fervently dispute attempts by some

CHAPTER 10

Christians to rationalize why God would use any bully as a divine instrument of gospel truth and might. I believe Jesus would agree with John Fea, a professor of evangelical history at Messiah College, who states that twisting the Bible in this way "is the theopolitical version of money laundering, taking Scripture to . . . clean [up] your candidate."[40]

Jesus brought a message of living with integrity, the divine action of love that has the power to bring the world into the peaceful balance God desires. This truth remains, no matter how twisted the rationalizations become to justify God using an oppressor to represent Christ and Christianity. Let God's grace as demonstrated through Jesus's integrity be the guide, for every person who calls themselves Christian or an admirer of Christ, for how we are to conduct our religious, political, and social lives.

To genuinely love Jesus, we need to appreciate the vital importance of honesty and respect in helping us to clearly see, predict, and prevent an outcome that gives ruthless people a voice, power, and influence. To honor Jesus, we demand his integrity from anyone who desires to hold a leadership role in our government.

For only when we share a mutual devotion to living aligned with integrity will we come together to find common ground based on truth, justice, and accountability.

11

United We Stand

As the saying goes, "United we stand; divided we fall."

Jesus was cooperative and respectful, and he stood for equity and social justice. He would want us to consider bipartisan government profoundly important. A collaborative, aware, and progressive Jesus would not want us to have blind allegiance to one side, one point of view, or the biased frenzy that comes from believing the candidate, party, or single issue we support has to prevail at all costs.

"Treat others as we want to be treated" applies to politics, too. And this brings us to an item of great importance in solving the "divided we fall" stalemate we often experience within our political system of government: the oath our elected public servants take establishes that they will work collaboratively to ensure the most effective, efficient, and successful legislation to advance our citizens and country forward to peace, equity, and unity.

Rather than be united on the common goals all citizens and leaders need to hold in order to preserve, progress, and defend our republic, however, we separate ourselves with blind party loyalty, obstructionism, and insensitivity to one another. We automatically negate people whose ideologies, party, and candidates differ from

CHAPTER 11

our own. We are passive, silent, or uninformed about the harmful policies we witness or champion (regarding women's rights or the LGBTQIA+ community, for example) because they don't personally threaten us. We don't want to admit that our indifferent response to the cries of the oppressed stems from our privilege of not being directly harmed by policies fueled by our self-centered political and religious agendas. Each of us has a responsibility to help protect the human rights of all citizens by being politically active and informed, yet we diminish the value of that responsibility.

We may justify our political passivity as not being required for our spirituality. We are wrong about this. We need to be talking about politics and religion in respectful and honest ways. We should have intelligent and bipartisan conversation. And we must be educated about the facts because being politically active is a spiritual responsibility.

Jesus did not separate his political action from his spirituality by playing the "politics is nonspiritual" card. Christ was a huge political and social activist for the abused and oppressed. In the words of Reverends Emily Swan and Ken Wilson, "The authors of the New Testament summon us to reject mimicking the crowd, and instead invite us to emulate Jesus."[41]

Doesn't it seem logical that Jesus would be disappointed that we have apathetically allowed our representative form of government to become a bitter contest between rival teams?

In November 2017, a citizen named David Fastenow wrote a letter to the editor of his local newspaper in Hot Springs, Arkansas. "I was traveling and came upon a group of people," he wrote. "I asked if I could join them, and they responded, Are you a Democrat or Republican? The question caught me off guard, as it did not used to matter."[42]

United We Stand

Why *does* political party affiliation matter?

Our democracy was not designed to divide us into opposing teams. We are citizens of a country founded upon the ideals of fairness. We are to share a commitment to the rule of law, to democracy, and to equal political, religious, and social rights. We are to be active participants in our shared civic life. We must be willing to sacrifice for the ideals we hold in common.

Although we have yet to live up to the goal of a common good, we must strive to continue to pursue the aspiration by walking the path of nonrivalry that Jesus encouraged. Which means each of us must call out those who scapegoat people they consider different and less than themselves. We must not turn a blind eye to those who oppress others. We must forcefully reject any claim by an oppressor or proven liar that they are the innocent one or they are the true victim.

We must value that our democracy was founded upon the ideals for all citizens to be on the same team when it comes to sharing core fundamental beliefs. Beliefs like everyone has the right to life, liberty, and the pursuit of happiness, no matter our gender, sexual orientation, religion, or skin color. Women and men are equal. Truth and fact matter as does a free press to hold those in power accountable. People who lie for whatever reason must be held accountable. There is no place for racism, bigotry, prejudice, or any form of discrimination. Diversity is a benefit. And peaceful protests in support of these beliefs are necessary to achieving and maintaining our freedom.

We, as equal citizens of the United States of America, must care to uphold these shared beliefs. We must defend them. To have a functioning society we must hold those we elect accountable to uphold and defend these shared common values too.

CHAPTER 11

You and I are responsible to an inclusive Jesus to call political party discord into question. George Washington, along with the other founders of our country, justifiably feared the likelihood of corruption and abuse of power that would arise from partisan divisiveness. They feared the tyranny of the majority. And, according to Max Boot, historian, best-selling author, and foreign-policy analyst, our country's founders also feared the tyranny of the minority. He writes,

> Everyone knows that the Founders were afraid of the tyranny of the majority. That's why they built so many checks and balances into the Constitution. What's less well known is that they were also afraid of the tyranny of the minority. In Federalist No. 22, Alexander Hamilton warned that giving small states like Rhode Island or Delaware "equal weight in the scale of power" with large states like "Massachusetts, or Connecticut, or New York" violated the precepts of "justice" and "common-sense." "The larger States would after a while revolt from the idea of receiving the law from the smaller," he predicted, arguing that such a system contradicts the fundamental maxim of republican government, which requires that the sense of the majority should prevail.
>
> Hamilton's nightmare has become the reality of 21st-century America. We are living under minoritarian tyranny, with smaller states imposing their views on the larger through their disproportionate sway in the Senate and the electoral college—and therefore on the Supreme Court. . . . We are experiencing what the Founders feared: a crisis of governmental legitimacy brought about by minoritarian tyranny.[43]

As citizens of a representative democracy and lovers of Christ, we must grasp that without valuing respect, solidarity, and balanced representation, politicians and citizens alike easily fall into a combative, self-interested, ego-boxing standstill.

Mickey Edwards, a member of Congress for sixteen years (1977–1993) and a former chairman of the House Republican leadership's Policy Committee, agrees it is vital we end partisanship. He says,

> If we are truly a democracy—if voters get to size up candidates for a public office and choose the one they want—why don't the elections seem to change anything? Because we elect our leaders, and they then govern, in a system that makes cooperation almost impossible and incivility nearly inevitable, a system in which the campaign season never ends and the struggle for party advantage trumps all other considerations.
>
> This is not an accident. Ours is a system focused not on collective problem-solving but on a struggle for power between two private organizations. Party activists control access to the ballot through closed party primaries and conventions; partisan leaders design congressional districts. Once elected to Congress, our representatives are divided into warring camps. Partisans decide what bills to take up, what witnesses to hear, what amendments to allow.
>
> Many Americans assume that's just how democracy works, that this is how it has always been, that it is the system the Founders created. But what we have today is a far cry from what the Founders intended. George Washington and James Madison both warned of the dangers posed by political parties. Defenders of the party system argue that parties—including Madison's own—arose almost immediately after the nation was founded. But those were not parties in the modern sense: they were factions uniting on a few

CHAPTER 11

major issues, not marching in lockstep on every issue, large and small. And while some defend the party system as a necessary provider of cues to voters who otherwise might not know how to vote, the Internet and mass media now make it possible for voters to educate themselves about candidates for office.[44]

Partisan politics is not servant leadership. Partisan politics does not lend itself to bettering our nation and the lives of our citizens. One-sidedness is void of the honesty and self-regulation necessary to overpower the egocentric motivation to rule and dominate. We need to realize those who are driven by the quest for power and dominance are not working for God or for us citizens but for themselves or those from whom they receive financial support.

Jesus would remind us that only leaders with empathy for all citizens are capable of working cooperatively to uphold the core social values of our democratic republic. I believe Jesus wants us to appreciate the actions of servant leaders who do work across the aisle. Therefore, you and I have the responsibility to be political by being informed so we can vote responsibly in every election—and that means up and down the ballot.

We cannot simply vote for the highest offices and expect our government to work efficiently and effectively. We have to care about selecting the right person for each position or measure on the ballot. We do our own investigation of the issues and candidates, and we don't listen to or are not influenced by attack ads, opinionated commentary, or uninformed relatives and friends. We are willing to cross the aisle to support women and men whose records represent the needs of their constituents. We do

United We Stand

everything within our power to refuse to give leadership positions to those who are comfortable with corruption, abuse of power, and the rewards of big business or money, or to those who vilify a free press that is vital to holding those in power accountable. We grow and change in positive ways by demanding greatness from ourselves and those we trust to represent us.

Yes, we can continue the dysfunction, partisanship, and constant fighting that are an unhealthy sign egocentric irresponsibility is very much in control in ourselves and in our government.

But is this the way we want our children to serve one another? Is this the system we want to pass on to future generations?

I believe Jesus would ask us to consider that in order to be a great nation, we have to value being governed by leaders Jesus would consider to be great—not "great" by the definition of a narrow, exclusionary view of Christian "rightness" but "great" in terms of living as he did, building relationships with people unlike himself in order to demonstrate compassion, kindness, and care for individuals and marginalized groups. Great leaders are those who, with consistent integrity and compassion, work for our citizenry as a whole. They don't have an "us against them" attitude. Great leaders value being on the same team, one that is dedicated to finding innovative solutions to the challenges we face.

To create positive, lasting change, we have to do something different. In the words (probably apocryphally) attributed to Albert Einstein, "The definition of insanity is doing the same thing over and over again and expecting different results." Regardless of who actually said it, the wisdom is sound and something we can follow to fix our broken system of government.

For instance, if we cannot see our way past clinging to our current two-party political system, let's at least think outside the

CHAPTER 11

box. Let's make a positive change in the organizational structure of government—one that supports cooperation, respect, and ethical oversight.

Why not consider electing copresidents, one from each of two major political parties?

They run on the same ticket against other nominees for copresident. They serve together and share power. No more same-party vice presidents. Let's get to the root of our two-party dissension and quests for power over one another by removing the built-in division, starting at the top and then creatively working our way down.

I know this may sound wild at first because it is so far outside of our long-standing method of governance, but surely it's at least worth considering. When I worked at Birmingham-Southern College, two of my bosses were the dean partners for graduate programs and the Division of Business. These two individuals of different genders, backgrounds, education, beliefs, and experience implemented a form of organizational leadership that took advantage of collaboration, shared responsibility, and diversity. Strategic thinking, decision-making, and unity were enriched through a team framework. They did not agree on everything. They agreed to disagree, agreeably, in order to arrive at solutions that were best for the organization as a whole. There were greatness and creativity in their cooperative relationship.

Of course, egotistic shortsightedness and desires for ruling power will say this copresident idea is impossible, ridiculous, not what our founders envisioned, or just plain nuts. There are many situations we face today that our founders did not predict, such as continuous war and prisons as businesses, or average citizens arming themselves with military-style weapons. However, they did foresee the threat of our democracy being overthrown by autocrats, dictators, and oligarchs. They feared the danger of dark money that buys influence and policy. They also wisely predicted the constant fighting, dishonesty, and abuses of power by career politicians who ignore their first and foremost duty to serve the public with honesty, cooperation, forethought, and respect.

Imagine the experience, diversity, and opportunity of truly balanced representation in government. Imagine how a focus on selecting people of truthfulness, with differing views yet common dedication to our democracy, would help eliminate the partisan war for power and money that results in influenced policy and political favors. What's wrong with exploring more creative solutions than the system we have now?

It may be time for us to begin ushering in a new form of government: *sortition democracy*, a system devised by ancient Athenians that taps into the wisdom of the crowd and entrusts ordinary people with making balanced decisions for the well-being of everyone.

In his book *The End of Politicians: Time for a Real Democracy*, Brett Hennig explores the random selection process in a sortition democracy that is run directly by many citizens rather than a few elected officials.[45] Chosen in a process similar to jury selection, these random citizens are drawn from a pool that is specifically designed to match the social and demographic profile of the citizenry, so they become an accurate representation of the population. This means 50 percent are women. A few would be wealthy, but the majority would be middle and lower income. Diverse ethnicity and sexual orientation would also represent the population as a whole.

The sortition democracy's random-selection process ensures government is not run by fringe public opinion, partisan politics, businesses, special-interest groups, career politicians, lobbyists, and money.

CHAPTER 11

In proposing these different ideas, I admit this is a complex issue. One vital change necessary to ensure our welfare as citizens is ending the practice of lobbyists rather than bipartisan experts providing data to Congress. We must understand, lobbying is a paid activity in which special interests hire well-connected, professional advocates to push specific legislation that benefits those who hire them. This type of biased activity happens at every level of government—local, state, and federal. The policies that often result from industry-specific legislation end up working in favor of those industries rather than the citizenry. And sometimes, former lobbyists are appointed to lead the federal or state agencies they once lobbied.

For example, an oil and gas or coal lobbyist has a vested interest in running the Environmental Protection Agency so they can enact policies that benefit the industry they were formerly paid to represent or eliminate policies that don't.

Similarly, rich and powerful people often exercise enormous influence over governmental officials. Robert Reich, retired Chancellor's Professor of Public Policy at the University of California at Berkeley, posed a question I bet the majority of us can't answer. I couldn't. He writes:

> Ever notice how there never seems to be enough money to build public infrastructure like mass transit lines and better schools? And yet, when a multi-billion-dollar sports team demands a new stadium, our local governments are happy to oblige. . . .
> It's part of a well established playbook. Billionaire buys a sports team.
> Billionaire pressures local government. Billionaire threatens to sell or move the team unless their demands are met.

United We Stand

Since 1990, franchises in major North American sports leagues have intercepted upwards of $30 billion worth of taxpayer funds from state and local governments to build stadiums. . . .

We, taxpayers, are essentially paying for the homes of our favorite sports teams, but we don't *really* own those homes, we don't get to rent them out, and we still have to buy expensive tickets to visit them.

Whenever these billionaire owners try to sell us on a shiny new stadium, they claim it will spur economic growth from which we'll all benefit. But numerous studies have shown that this is false.

As a University of Chicago economist aptly put it, "If you want to inject money into the local economy, it would be better to drop it from a helicopter than invest it in a new ballpark."

But what makes sports teams special is they are one of the few realms of collective identity we have left.

Billionaires prey on the love that millions of fans have for their favorite teams. . . .

We are underfunding public necessities in order to funnel money to billionaires for something they could feasibly afford.[46]

Shouldn't we consider schemes like this a legal form of extortion and bribery? Don't we need to confront honestly the seriousness of money rather than morals being in control of our government? Does it not seem likely that Jesus would say financial power must never outdo our self-governing power?

Removing dark money that buys influence, power, and policy—including that from foreign governments—is a huge piece

CHAPTER 11

of this complicated puzzle. We have to put an end to political spending by organizations that have been granted nonprofit status as a social organization, union, or trade association that are not required to disclose their donors. These types of organizations can receive unlimited contributions from individuals, unions, and corporations, with which they can influence elections to ensure the candidate(s) who support their self-serving agendas are elected. Or they use their influence and wealth to push a specific religious ideology.

For example, do we really believe Jesus would want to be associated with the Servant Foundation (behind the "He Gets Us" 2023 Superbowl ads about Jesus) when the nonprofit donated tens of millions to the Alliance Defending Freedom (ADF), a conservative anti-LGBTQ and anti-abortion organization that is labeled as a hate group by the Southern Poverty Law Center?[47]

In addition to removing dark money from the political process and religion, we need to secure our elections by providing federal assistance to states to improve and safeguard their election systems. And we must restore the most important part of our democracy: the guarantee that every citizen has safe and easy access to voting.

This means we remove such obstacles as voter suppression and discrimination. We make voting easy. We have a national holiday on Election Day so people are not forced to miss work in order to stand in line to cast their ballot.

These are hardly radical suggestions. Shouldn't we be skeptical of the motivation of any political party, leader, or Supreme Court Justice who is opposed to fair and equal access to voting? Ensuring accessible and fair elections must be entirely bipartisan.

In addition, let's become educated about the civic duty each citizen has to maintain the values of our democracy. Let's demand rigorous courses in civic education as a requirement for every middle- and high-school student—learning not just facts about the branches of government but also the practical aspects of being a citizen, including their rights and duties. We have to ensure that all citizens know the institutions, principles, and processes of government and that they appreciate the core ideas and shared values of our representative democracy. Education is key to creating a sense of belonging. Let's educate *ourselves* to the fact that we are limiting the effectiveness of any administration by forcing it to constantly campaign rather than allow it to concentrate on the job of representing us.

The largest piece that needs to fall into place to reform our government is demanding integrity and empathy from ourselves and those we elect to serve us. Regardless of what new management system we may implement to improve our government and society, we need to appreciate that in order to get different results, we need to do something radically different from what we are currently doing. In addressing any challenge we face, we must not allow ourselves to fall victim to a failure of imagination. We have to act to overcome our apathy in order to create real, lasting, positive change.

To create a future we are proud to leave to our children and theirs, the time has come to transform the structure of our society. Doing so requires us to rethink our political system. We must be informed and stay active, as Jesus would. We must view being involved in our political process and bettering society in general as core values and standard practices. We must also teach children to consider it part of their spiritual duty to demonstrate social responsibility and political awareness.

No matter what actions we take, we first must choose trustworthy leaders whose consistent actions reveal their dedication to truthfulness and inclusion. We have to admit that those who

CHAPTER 11

abuse power will readily abuse humanity; when those at the top establish what is best for all, there is a huge humanitarian cost. We need to understand those who buy influence in our government don't care about what is best for the citizens of our country. They are pressing a personal agenda that benefits themselves or the interests of their supporters. Therefore, we have to agree we cannot continue to divide ourselves as though government is a contest between rival teams.

Party label is unimportant to the health of our country. As citizens of a democratic republic, we are to be united and on the same team. That means we are obliged to come together in the common goal of valuing honesty and responsibility in ourselves and all of our public servants.

I don't believe an integrity-first public servant, collaborative administrator, or random-citizen-selection approach is naive. True superheroes are everyday people who strive to make the world a better place by adhering to the values of principled character. Great leaders find innovative solutions to the challenges they face. Consequently, the path to ushering in a new and workable way to govern our democracy will become clear once we place utmost importance on the conscientiousness of those we choose to fill leadership positions.

Whenever we are in doubt regarding a decision about whom Jesus would consider a great leader and public servant, let's envision him standing in front of us, looking us in the eye, and asking these questions:

- Are they cooperative?
- Do they behave with accountability?
- Do they, above all else, defend our constitutional democracy

(as an ever-changing work in progress) and work to protect the human rights of all citizens?
- Do they believe behaving with honesty is always the right thing to do?
- Are their education and experience adequate for the position?
- Do they welcome the personal and professional scrutiny of public service?
- Do they voluntarily submit to and pass thorough background checks, including providing their tax returns?
- Are they humble?
- Are they devoted to seeking cooperative solutions to challenges?
- Are they mindful, intelligent, and respectful?
- Are their decisions and comments fact- and evidence-based?
- Do you trust them with your children's social and environmental future?
- Do they stand for justice, gender equity, and the other values of respect?
- Are they willing to lead us in making amends for our history of abusing one another rather than intentionally attempt to suppress it?
- What have they done to promote peace, cooperation, and truthfulness?

To ensure we are part of the solution to keep our country moving toward a more perfect union, we must select leaders who will help us usher in a new era of unity. We must support leaders Jesus would support. United we will stand, and divided we will fall.

12

Racism, It's Time for Our Come-to-Jesus Moment

Picture the scene: Victoria, Texas, 1961. I am five years old, and my mom is taking me trick-or-treating at the home of a woman she knows.

Mom rings the doorbell, and Mrs. Lilly answers, smiling at my scary little costume as she puts several pieces of candy into my bag.

As we stand on the porch, a car pulls up to the curb and a little girl about my age, dressed like a witch, gets out of the back seat and begins walking up toward the porch toward us.

Mrs. Lilly pushes me aside as she lunges down the steps toward the girl. Stopping in the middle of the sidewalk, she plants her hands firmly on her hips, leans forward, and screams: "GET BACK IN THE CAR, N----R. I DON'T WANT YOU COMING UP HERE. GO BACK WHERE YOU BELONG!"

The evil energy of the old woman's hatred boomerangs back, hitting me square in the chest with such force I feel as if my heart might shatter. I can see from the girl's stunned look her heart is breaking, too, as the tears begin streaming down her cheeks. Certainly, this was not the first time a Black girl in 1960s Texas encountered such an attitude, but for this kind of bigoted hate to land on her in the middle of a lighthearted childhood ritual must have felt like a full-fisted gut punch to her innocence.

Silent, dejected, deflated, the little girl turned and got back in the car. I watched as the car pulled away. To this day I think of her. I can never banish the memory of witnessing hate hurled at another human being by someone who claimed to love God. Someone who went to church, sat in the pew each Sunday, and professed to love Jesus. Yet someone who did not, it seems, know much about Jesus, the dark-skinned, loving man who was not White, blue-eyed, blond, or Christian.[48]

Can we imagine how deeply God loved the soul we call Jesus—who was not in the body of a White man? *How would it feel to a dark-skinned Jesus to hear us say the N-word?*

As a first-century Eastern Mediterranean man of Jewish descent, Jesus was not White. The White image we have of Jesus was created for us over time. We have passed on an inaccurate image of him, to the detriment of our human interactions.

Growing up in the American South during the 1960s, I was surrounded by ethnic tension, inequity, prejudice, bigotry, racism, and violence, perpetuated by people who claimed to love Jesus. Even as a child, I questioned the hypocrisy of those who believed they were entitled, in the name of their God, to treat *any* fellow human beings as less than themselves.

The exclusive and illogical belief that God created all human beings but somehow deemed light-skinned Christians better requires us to consider: *How would a Jewish, dark-skinned Jesus be treated in a world where White people walk through life unconcerned about their skin color, while their Brown and Black brothers and sisters don't have this freedom?*

White people *must* acknowledge White privilege. There was a time when I, as a White woman, walked through life unaware

CHAPTER 12

of the vast benefits provided to me simply because of my skin color—not being tailed by retail workers or security when I shop, not having to worry about excessive force in a routine traffic stop, people automatically assuming I have a college degree because of how I look. I am no longer unaware of the advantages of my White skin, but I still don't know what it is like for my sisters and brothers with darker skin. That is why I asked four of my friends of color to provide a glimpse into the world in which they grew up and still live in today for any readers who might need some context.

In my friend Shanti's June 18, 2019, email to me she wrote:

> The teacher touched Barbara's hair reverently as she glared at me with disgust. "This is how clean hair is supposed to look!" Her scorn cut like a knife.
>
> Although I was only in the third grade at my private Catholic school, I understood the message. I wasn't the right anything. Color, shape, hair length and texture. I knew it, because every time I had to stand in front of the class and say my name, my stomach lurched up into my throat. I felt I would be sick at being so vulnerably exposed as different.
>
> Growing up, I wasn't allowed to have friends. No birthday parties, sleepovers, or after-school get-togethers. This didn't make the dark-haired, tan-skinned Puerto Rican-and-Indian girl very popular in the mostly Eastern European Ridgewood neighborhood between Brooklyn and Queens, New York. Life was very difficult. Being chased home at least three times a week by a group of white girls. Called "nigger" and "spic."
>
> I understood not being liked for my personality or actions. But to have such disdain for my color, culture, or ethnicity just never made sense to me, since I couldn't control those aspects of myself even if I wanted to.

Racism, It's Time for Our Come-to-Jesus Moment

I hold no animosity or antagonism for people who judge and put me down. I understand this is what has been taught, so it is their default setting. I always felt Jesus loved me no matter if my skin was darker compared to my classmates. It never mattered to him, and perhaps that's why I am devoted to help Jesus love the world as it seems a huge job for one man.

Shanti is correct that loving the world is a huge job for one man or woman. We also agree that in order to honor Jesus, we need to be aware that White privilege and supremacy continue, as they have for centuries, to infect our attitudes and treatment of one another.

Prejudicial and bigoted beliefs influence more than just the attitudes of White people. As my friend Crissy, in a June 3, 2019, email, explains:

My experience with white supremacy and white privilege is somewhat different. Growing up African American in Birmingham, Alabama, it was commonplace for there to be tension of some sort between people of different races, religions, and preferences of any kind. But my issue growing up Black was not so much suffering ill treatment from people who were different from me. It was being discriminated against for not being Black enough by people who looked like me.

My mother was referred to by the Black community as "paper-sack brown." Hours after my birth, my paternal grandfather questioned my legitimacy, as he said no one in their family was that "bright." Growing up, I experienced unjust judgment and isolation because of the complexion of my skin, which caused me to question why I wasn't darker, since

CHAPTER 12

the people I loved and admired had deep melanin and were beautiful and regal, in my opinion. This was a problem for me, because my cousins thought our grandmother loved me more because I had a lighter complexion. Classmates said my Caucasian teachers treated me better because I was almost white. Even the person who would become my best friend initially didn't care much for me. Because I was light skinned, she assumed I thought I was better than everyone else.

Ultimately, what helped me deal with being a light-skinned Black girl was being taught God made me exactly as God wants me to be. Anyone who has a problem with me, then, has a problem with God. No matter how I was treated by members of my own community, I was taught not to judge a person by anything other than their character. My grandmother always said, "Let people be who they are! We don't have a Heaven or Hell to put them in!"

I've learned people who discriminate against others or attempt to make them feel uncomfortable, for whatever reason, don't take time to get to know them. When we do take time to get to know who someone is beyond skin color, more often than not we find most people have hearts of gold.

I agree with Crissy: many people have a heart of gold. But too many of us don't do what we know Jesus would do because we succumb to peer pressure. People who truly honor Jesus separate themselves from the misguided crowd.

These beliefs are certainly not correct in the eyes of God, who created all of us and who sent a loving soul in the body of a dark-skinned Jesus to show us what it means to love one another. Jesus taught that our true value to God is measured by the integrity of our character. Our integrity is determined by whether we treat

Racism, It's Time for Our Come-to-Jesus Moment

people respectfully, without excuses, justifications, or using misguided and hurtful beliefs as weapons against one another. These are negative experiences my friend Sharmila knows well. She says in a May 28, 2019, email,

> From as early as I remember, I was made to believe that the lightness of one's skin determined the person's value. Since I was born with caramel-color skin, I would have to make myself as unobtrusive as possible in order to win at the game of life.
>
> Growing up in the 1980s on the outskirts of Indianapolis, Indiana, I was unusual, not only as a child of Indian immigrants, but because both my mom and dad worked outside the home. There were very few after-school programs my family could afford. This is how my Hindu parents ended up sending my brother and me to a local Christian academy. I don't have many fond memories of my time there.
>
> When I was about six years old, I remember standing at one of the school's drinking fountains sipping water. A group of boys taunted me with shouts of "Big Lips" and called me the N-word. I was called the N-word a lot.
>
> But the most upsetting memory I have of my time at the Christian academy was the day in Bible class when we were told Jesus hates people who don't believe in him. I asked the teacher, "What about my parents? They are Hindu, they don't believe in Jesus—but they are good people, what about them?"
>
> I will never forget the teacher's cruel response: "Your parents are going to Hell."
>
> As an adult, I know the hatred, the judgmental teachings I received, and the verbal abuse by those boys were all mo-

CHAPTER 12

tivated by their belief white was right and better. They were taught to be scared of the unfamiliar.

I now am blessed to know the most amazing Christians. They are people who live the true meaning of the word "Christian." I also know incredible Hindus, Muslims, Jews, Buddhists, atheists, Wiccans—people of all, any, and no religions. All of these loving and accepting people believe all life is precious. They all believe love is love. And no matter how much I was and might still be hated by some for my beautiful caramel-color skin, to me love is the most important religion of all.

Christianity must motivate only Christlike inclusion of difference. What would Jesus think about people who use the religion founded in his name to persecute anyone?

I hope we can all agree defending hate, persecution, and suppression of people in God's name is not of God, no matter the religious identification or justification. Surely, a quarter of the way through the twenty-first century, we can all agree that discrimination based on the way a person was created by God is wrong. To honor God, we remember the Golden Rule is the foundation of all world religions. No matter how we worship God, the goal of all spiritual practice is to treat people as we want to be treated. That means everyone, not just those who look like us and believe as we do. The Golden Rule commands us to honor the experiences of the oppressed and protect them as Jesus did.

To achieve the goal of living by the Golden Rule, we need to accept that valuing "White" or "Christian" to the detriment of others who also belong to God's beautiful tapestry of human beings is an egocentric practice deeply entrenched in our social, political, and religious lives. We need to realize these divisive and

Racism, It's Time for Our Come-to-Jesus Moment

destructive beliefs are deep-rooted in our history and continue to be taught to children in both subtle and overt ways.

My friend Miguel shared with me in a June 18, 2019, email his experience of being trained by those around him to believe he was less than people whose skin was White:

> It is my experience that when most people speak of issues concerning White supremacy, they are thinking of overt, blatant acts of racism, like racial slurs and KKK rallies. They are not thinking of the more common, subtle, and casual manifestations many People of Color call "polite" White supremacy.
>
> Growing up, I can't say I remember being disrespected often with blatant racial slurs. But what I did start noticing at a very young age was the preference for Whiteness, whether it was noticing that every "truly successful" person exalted in society was White, or noticing Mexican parents training their children to appease the comfort levels and preferences of White folks. The subliminal, suggested message in media and society was that we should be as White as possible. This is even so in Mexican society, where Spanish-European aesthetics and the Catholic religion are venerated and anything denoting indigeneity is disparaged. "Kill the Indian—Save the Man," as the sentiment goes.
>
> Superman and Batman were White, as were all the American heroes saving the world in Hollywood movies. My social reality showed that most Mexicans were poor, in a gang, or in jail. Of course, as a child I witnessed all of these dynamics with zero knowledge of self or the historical contexts to my thoughts, such as "Why are Mexicans poor and in jail and White people rich and successful?"

CHAPTER 12

As a child, you're not critical of these subliminal factors of White supremacy, but the inferred messages implant a sense of hate for anything about yourself that doesn't fit White society. Even now, my peers sometimes put pressure on me—a grown man—to "tone down" my truth-based perspectives of racism, thus continuing the domesticated habit of conceding to White fragility at the expense of the voices of People of Color who seek justice and healing.

Miguel and all of my Brown and Black friends respect what I go through as a gay person who is frequently persecuted and dehumanized for my sexual orientation. They also accept that I, as a White woman, have no real understanding of their experiences of moving through life as people of color. They appreciate that I don't pretend that our experiences are the same.

It is important that White people acknowledge that most people—including Black, Brown, and White—were taught an inaccurate version of our shared history, one that was intentionally crafted by multiple generations of White European Americans in an attempt to relieve their cognitive dissonance over the horrors they committed against people of color. White people need to own the part their White ancestors played in that mistreatment. White people need to accept that the playing field was never, and still isn't, fair here in America. We need to wrestle with the sad truth that White skin continues to provide advantages within American society, even without the realization or consent of White people. We need to grow our awareness about how we must help move our society toward equality by speaking up against White supremacy and privilege.

White people who love Jesus and God must come together to act on behalf of sisters and brothers of every race. In the words of Debby Irving,

Racism, It's Time for Our Come-to-Jesus Moment

How can racism possibly be dismantled until white people, lots and lots of white people, understand it as an unfair system, get in touch with the subtle stories and stereotypes that play in their heads, and see themselves not as good or bad but as players in the system? Until white people embrace the problem, the elephant in the room—and all the nasty tension and mistrust that go with it—will endure. And the feedback efforts of people of color will fall on ignorant ears at best, or be misconstrued as too whiney or too angry at worst.[49]

To begin healing, we must agree that no matter our skin color, gender, sexual orientation, or religion, what is most important is that we respect one another. We agree the solution to judgment, condemnation, and the injustices committed because of our differences is establishing empathy, so we can see ourselves in each other. After all, *wouldn't Jesus find our lack of respect for one another disappointing, after we've had thousands of years to get this aspect of his integrity right?*

First, let's take a closer look at the definition of racism as it differs from prejudice and bigotry.

Debby Irving writes:

Prejudice is when a person negatively pre-judges another person or group without getting to know the beliefs, thoughts, and feelings behind their words and actions. A person of any racial group can be prejudiced towards a person of any other racial group. There is no power dynamic involved.

Bigotry is stronger than prejudice, a more severe mindset and often accompanied by discriminatory behavior. It's arrogant and mean-spirited, but requires neither systems nor power to engage in.

CHAPTER 12

Racism is the system that allows the racial group that's already in power to retain power. Since arriving on U.S. soil white people have used their power to create preferential access to survival rights and resources (housing, education, jobs, voting, citizenship, food, health, legal protection, etc.) for white people while simultaneously impeding people of color's access to these same rights and resources. Though "reverse racism" is a term I sometimes hear, it has never existed in America. White people are the only racial group to have ever established and retained power in the United States.[50]

Racism appears, for example, in the intolerance behind replacement theory. Pushed by on-air infotainment personalities, politicians, and right-wing conspiracy theorists, this is the idea that White people are being intentionally "replaced" by Black and Brown people, Jews, Muslims, or various immigrant groups— and this idea fans the flames of fear and hatred. The people who promote this idea consider themselves patriots devoted to the United States, yet they seem to overlook the fact that ours is a nation founded by immigrants. And what's more, it was established on land stolen from indigenous people who were systematically murdered and abused.

Jesus would challenge us, as a supposedly Christ-loving nation, to get on the same page about the fundamental mission of this country. In the words of the forty-third President of the United States, Republican George W. Bush, "Our identity as a nation, unlike other nations, is not determined by geography or ethnicity, by soil or blood. . . . This means that people of every race, religion, and ethnicity can be fully and equally American. It means that bigotry or White supremacy in any form is blasphemy against the American creed."[51]

Racism, It's Time for Our Come-to-Jesus Moment

Racism was historically fueled by many legalized, codified factors, such as the religious justifications for slavery and the fact that the crafters of the Constitution permitted that enslaved people count as only three-fifths of a human for census-taking purposes.[52] Prejudice is found in the lack of Black- and Brown-authored books that are required reading for high-school and college courses—and in the number of them currently on various public-school-library "banned" lists.

White readers may be thinking, "Of course slavery was bad, but no one actually believes this stuff anymore. I don't mind sharing a drinking fountain with Black people; doesn't that show I've done the work?" If that is you, please allow me to ask this: were you taught to believe people of color are less than people who are White?

I was.

I was taught a distorted portrayal of enslavement as a happy existence in which enslaved people sang joyfully while they worked in the fields and elsewhere. I was taught that people in human bondage learned vital skills, so it was ultimately a beneficial system for them; some children today are still being taught that.[53] Today, many people want to bury the real horrors of daily life for those Black enslaved human beings, including the rampant beatings, murders, and violent rape of women and girls.

Many White people also discount the horrors of the thousands of lynchings that took place after slavery ended. These murders were viewed as a justified response to the fear White people had of formerly enslaved people. These fears fueled years of institutionalized subjugation through the enactment of Black codes and Jim Crow laws. Replacement theory is not a new trend.

Today, in some parts of the southern United States, the Civil War is still referred to as the "War of Northern Aggression." As Mashama Bailey writes,

CHAPTER 12

The reprehensible part of this conversation is that they are not talking about how horrible and inhumane slavery was or how the North came down and righted this wrong. They are still talking about how the North came down and fucked up their shit. Why don't they start talking about the division between classes, which is just a euphemism for "race" in the South, and how it is so damned stark that there is a pervasive hopelessness in it all? Because, I think they like it like that. The sad part is that the line of division is literally right in front of our faces. You can look to the other side of the street and see how badly people are living and yet the people who are supposed to lead change don't seem to be affected by seeing it.[54]

The continued violations of human rights and the intentional suppression of people of color are a result of a system of inaccurate and absurd beliefs, behaviors, and fears. This system spawns racism visible in employment and housing discrimination; in urban planning; in city, state, and federal policies; in higher interest rates for people with darker skin; in people of color being too often wrongly accused and thrown in jail without access to adequate legal counsel or justice. And the violations continue, as God knows: mass incarceration. Food deserts. Generational poverty. Worse air quality than in White communities. Less access to health care than White people. Generational stress. Racist mascots. The Confederate flag. Confederate statues. Columbus Day celebrations. Anti-immigration policies and practices. Victim blaming. Police brutality. White supremacy. Manifest destiny.

Joy DeGruy writes,

> Americans are socialized to believe in the American dream. They are socialized to believe that America is the land of

Racism, It's Time for Our Come-to-Jesus Moment

opportunity, a land in which anyone can, with hard work and ingenuity, accomplish anything, a land in which even a person from the poorest of backgrounds can one day grow up to be president. They are socialized to believe they live in a country in which the ideals of equality, liberty, and justice for all reign supreme. They are socialized to believe America is the best country in the world and that Americans are the best people. Most Americans believe themselves to be the most caring, most just, most industrious, and most generous people in the world.

And most Americans are socialized to believe that white is better. It's better than yellow; it's better than red; it's better than light brown, and it's much better than dark brown. The poorest, most ignorant, ill-tempered white person still believes him- or herself to be better than anyone not white.[55]

These words from Dr. DeGruy make me wonder: to honor Jesus, don't we need to assume responsibility for the injustices that were and continue to be committed against our fellow human beings?

Don't we need to individually and collectively admit the playing field was never level?

Don't we need to face the fact that those too often viewed as not working hard enough to achieve the American dream were cheated out of it in the first place?

Debby Irving clarifies some of the history it is essential that White people learn and acknowledge:

Between 1934 and 1962 the federal government underwrote $120 billion in new housing, less than 2 percent of which went to people of color. America's largest single investment

CHAPTER 12

in its people, through an intertwined structure of housing and banking systems, gave whites a lifestyle and financial boost that would accrue in the decades to come while driving Blacks and other minority populations into a downward spiral. Discriminatory practices among colleges, universities, banks, and realtors created an impenetrable barrier to the GI Bill's promise, turning America's golden opportunity to right its racially imbalanced ship into an acceleration of its listing. From the perspective of Americans excluded from this massive leg-up policy, home loans and the GI Bill are two examples of affirmative action for white people.[56]

This gross and deliberate inequity is illustrated very clearly in the instances Irving cites, but we all know that those were not anomalies from an otherwise stellar pattern of equal treatment. As Michelle Alexander documents,

> In each generation, new tactics have been used for achieving the same goals—goals shared by the Founding Fathers. Denying African Americans citizenship was deemed essential to the formation of the original union. Hundreds of years later, America is still not an egalitarian democracy. The arguments and rationalizations that have been trotted out in support of racial exclusion and discrimination in its various forms have changed and evolved, but the outcome has remained largely the same.
>
> What has changed since the collapse of Jim Crow has less to do with the basic structure of our society than with the language we use to justify it. In the era of colorblindness, it is no longer socially permissible to use race, explicitly, as a justification for discrimination, exclusion, and social contempt.

Racism, It's Time for Our Come-to-Jesus Moment

So we don't. Rather than rely on race, we use our criminal justice system to label people of color "criminals" and then engage in all the practices we supposedly left behind.[57]

This ought to make us wonder: do we want to look Jesus in the eye and justify a society where hatred, prejudice, and abuse are tolerated or defended?

Don't we need to admit ego's drive to feel superior over those we deem inferior comes at a great personal, social, and spiritual cost?

Don't we honor Jesus by righting the wrongs of injustice?

It's simple—God created all human beings as equal. To honor Jesus, we cannot allow those who abandon fact, human decency, and respect for all life to justify their actions as "White supremacy." The belief that ethnic or religious dominance is necessary in order to establish and maintain a productive and safe society is not aligned with God, who created all life. This fear-based motivation for control does not come from a heart that reflects the inclusive values Jesus held dear. He would remind us that our value as members of the human family is determined by how we treat all people. He would ask us to value respect over disrespect, kindness above cruelty, and justice over injustice.

White people who say they love Jesus have to admit they must do more to end their own racial dominance, just as they must do more to end male dominance over women. Many White people find the injustices of White privilege and systemic racism intolerable. White people owe it to a dark-skinned Jesus not only to acknowledge that the dehumanization of people of color continues within society but to denounce it loudly. White people must be careful not to center themselves in this work and must do everything within their power to end it for their children and

CHAPTER 12

their children's children. It requires them to be a role model so those who follow view people of all ethnicities as true equals. And it requires White people to humble themselves to listen to what is being asked of them from communities of color rather than sweeping in and imposing their own ideas to "magically fix" what is broken.

We must be willing to speak up against racism in daily life and work to dismantle imbalanced systems and rebuild them fairly. We must encourage those in our workplaces to recruit and promote qualified people of color and pay them the same as their White counterparts. We need to believe people when they call out racism, just as we need to believe those who reveal experiences of sexual abuse.

We must demand police accountability. At the same time, we must ease the burden police currently bear to handle situations they are not trained to deal with. This will require reallocating funds to mental health, homelessness, affordable housing, education, and other social initiatives that help communities thrive.

We must vigorously work to level the playing field among Americans of all races, such as by increasing funding for financial and educational programs that positively affect people of color.

And we must accept our history. While we cannot change the past, we can and must work hard to change our future. We do so through honest conversations and by demanding that all children be taught an accurate history of enslavement in the Western world. We become informed by reading books such as Elie Mystal's *Allow Me to Retort: A Black Guy's Guide to the Constitution* and *The 1619 Project: A New Origin Story* edited by Nikole Hannah-Jones, Caitlin Roper, Ilena Silverman, and Jake Silverstein.[58] In addition, we become—and stay—aware of how advertising, entertainment, media, housing, laws, employment and

Racism, It's Time for Our Come-to-Jesus Moment

educational opportunities, lending, and so much more are biased toward Whites. We open our hearts to the fact that too much of what is considered "legal" is not necessarily "moral" if it comes at someone's expense.

We remember Jesus's request to love our neighbor as ourselves because God created all of us as equals.

13

We Are Part of God's Big Family

Jean and Reagan Cates were unable to have children of their own, so they adopted me. Mom shared the memory of bringing me home from central to south Texas on an airplane: "I carried you on a newly purchased pillow in a plane full of curious strangers. I hoped against hope you wouldn't break before I got to your grandmother's house, where we stayed for several days while Dad moved us into the little house on Mistletoe Street. We just purchased the house right before we got the call about you. I remember clearly that you did not enjoy the airplane trip!"

I feel incredibly blessed my mother shared this memory with me. Although we have been through some hard times, we have created many more wonderful memories over the years. Mom and Dad are now two of my biggest fans and best friends and came to a place of unconditional love for me after bravely confronting their own beliefs about human sexuality.

But being adopted means there is also a birth mother and a story we share, too, no matter how brief.

On the one occasion my biological mother and I met, I learned she had turned fourteen right before I was born. As hard as it is to believe, she had not known she was pregnant. It was only after complaining of painful cramps that she was rushed to the hospital.

Three days after I was born, she decided to give me up for adoption. However, the religious guilt and persecution she faced over premarital sex and unwed pregnancy forced her to marry my biological father. Over time, they had four more children, my full biological brothers and sisters.

After years of fantasizing about how it would be to meet my biological mother, I finally reached out when I was twenty-one. I was able to find her because the adoption had been arranged by a physician who was a relative of my adoptive mother, Jean. He kept in touch with my birth mother, Mary, and knew where to find her should I ever want to connect. I did, and we made a plan.

As you can imagine, I was excited to meet her and my biological brothers and sisters. My adoptive parents, Jean and Reagan, were happy for me, too. They were not envious because they considered this meeting an opportunity for more people to love me. But sadly, that was not what happened.

The day I spent with them was extremely unpleasant. When I told them I was gay, they slammed the door shut on having a relationship with me. My birth mother did not allow my biological siblings to have anything to do with me.

I had never met these people before, so I was not completely devastated by their cruel rejection. By the time I connected with them, I had already endured substantial religious persecution and suffering for being different, so that was nothing new. But I don't consider being accustomed to hatred and discrimination a badge of honor. As a gay person growing up in a Christian church, I was aware early in life how much some people despise difference, in any form.

CHAPTER 13

Since I was adopted three days after my birth and rejected by my biological family before I could ask many questions, I knew nothing about my heritage. To find out about my ancestors, I did a DNA test and learned some of my ancestors were not White. In fact, I am related to "Cheddar man," a fossil unearthed in 1903 in Gough's Cave, located in Somerset's Cheddar Gorge, England. Thanks to leading-edge scientific analysis, we now know my very distant relative lived around ten thousand years ago and had dark brown skin and blue eyes.

I have another ancestor who lived between 1690 and 1780 who was a Black West African, and another who lived in the early 1800s was Native American. Rounding out my DNA ancestors are people who were Iberian, Balkan, Irish, English, French, German, and Scandinavian. I carry within my own body a beautifully complex map of human diversity.

I am considered White, yet my DNA proves I am a combination of the colors and cultures of my ancestors. I am as proud of my dark-skinned genetic relatives as I am of my light-skinned ones.

Maybe you discovered some surprises in your own DNA after taking a test. Maybe you learned, as I did, about whole new facets of your family history you never even suspected. Or maybe you learned that you are 100 percent one racial group or another, with a pretty much direct, insular line over hundreds or even thousands of years. My point is this: our biological place in human history is fascinating, curious, *and totally out of our control*. Isn't it logical and responsible to admit that we, as a species, made up our "race problem"?

In *The Biology of Race*, James King writes: "Race is a concept of society that insists there is a genetic difference behind human variations in skin color that transcends outward appearance.

We Are Part of God's Big Family

However, race has no scientific merit outside of sociological classifications. There are no significant genetic variations within the human species to justify the division of 'races.'"[59]

Our problem is that we say God made all human beings equal, but we don't actually respect this fact. Egocentric quests for dominance and control over other people have fueled the long history of persecution of difference, including rigged rules against Black and Brown communities as well as discrimination against Asians, women, members of the LGBTQIA+ community, people with disabilities, and so forth. This means, no matter what we might like to say, we have a huge problem with God's grand design of genetic and biological diversity.

We don't respect one another's strengths, experiences, and life struggles. We lack respect for our differences. Respect for our shared humanity. Respect for the idea that we are to look for the good in one another and treat each person as we want to be treated—as the God-created soul we are. But wouldn't Jesus want us to acknowledge that respect is the foundation upon which all healthy relationships are based?

All of us who claim to love Jesus need to confront what we think we know about ourselves as a human family. We need to challenge what we have been programmed to believe about history. We seek to educate ourselves to the truth about how many Christians continue to support a system of misinformation, injustice, and the abuse of people of color. We acknowledge and teach all children the truth about the history of enslaving other human beings, Black codes, lynchings, unethical medical experimentation, and grossly unequal treatment in almost every aspect of society.

We confront the continuing brutality perpetrated by too many within the ranks of those who are charged with protecting and serving all of us. We admit that the toll of hundreds of years

CHAPTER 13

of physical and psychological torture inflicted on our brothers and sisters of different racial or ethnic groups will not simply "go away." We cannot allow ourselves or our politicians to dismiss honest discussion about our shared history with belittling statements such as "no one is being held in enslavement today, so just get over it." How arrogant, cruel, and insulting to our fellow human beings for anyone to want to move past our country's great White sin without owning it and making amends.

The fact is, deep cultural trauma does not simply disappear just because the people primarily affected have passed away. The trauma of racism is passed from generation to generation. Joy DeGruy reminds us: "African Americans have a unique socialization experience due to centuries of systematic and traumatic programming of inferiority, covering all aspects of one's being. In other words, from the beginning Africans were taught they were inferior physically, emotionally, intellectually, and spiritually, thus rendering them completely ineffectual in their own eyes and in the eyes of the society around them."[60]

To begin our collective healing, we accept that developments in human evolutionary genetics repudiate the myth of racial difference proposed by those who desire to promote White supremacy. For example, dark skin is more effective at sun protection, while light skin is better at making more vitamin D using less sunlight.[61] Different groups' skin pigment changed over thousands of years due to their migration patterns and how they processed vitamin D as they migrated out of Africa to populate the planet. This is simple science, not some divine mark of favor.

Still, there are those who insist otherwise, forcing us to ask the question: how would our human history be different if we had never fashioned Jesus into the inaccurate image of a White man?

We Are Part of God's Big Family

Others will insist the so-called Aryan race is genetically superior and therefore permitted by God to persecute the Jewish people. Conveniently ignoring the fact that Jesus was a Jew, for two millennia Christianity has portrayed Jews as the murderers of Jesus, even though he was executed under Pontius Pilate according to Roman (read: European) practice.

I know it is challenging to admit that many of us have been intentionally misinformed and misled about Jesus's skin color in traditions going back hundreds of years. It is not comfortable for White people to assume responsibility for the injustices our ancestors perpetuated throughout history on dark-skinned people. It is not easy to admit that those injustices still occur or that people still commit acts of antisemitism in Jesus's name. And it can be dangerous to stand up to those whose fear of losing professed dominance fuels their hateful, hurtful, and unjust treatment of people. But it is the duty of all Christians to love Jesus and to model our love on that of Jesus, who loved all equally.

True Jesus-respecting people have to be exceedingly brave. We stand up against abuses of authority and power. We care about the wrongs committed against other people. We do everything we can to make them right—even when doing so scares us.

Didn't Jesus bravely stand up to injustice?

Wouldn't a true friend of Jesus do the same?

When I lived in Birmingham, Alabama, in the early 1980s, I had a friend named Petric Smith who was faced with the reality that his uncle and three other Ku Klux Klansmen and segregationists planted at least fifteen sticks of dynamite beneath the front steps of the African American Sixteenth Street Baptist Church in Birmingham. The bombing on Sunday, September 15, 1963, when Petric (born Elizabeth Ann Hollifield) was twenty-three, killed four little girls; it was an act of White supremacist

CHAPTER 13

terrorism. In 1965, the Federal Bureau of Investigation concluded the church bombing had been committed by four known Klansmen. No prosecutions ensued until 1977, when Robert Chambliss, my friend's uncle, was tried and convicted of first-degree murder of one of the victims.

My friend was the star witness for the prosecution. Chambliss was convicted, in large part, as a result of Libby's testimony. After the trial, threats and harassment from Ku Klux Klan members forced Libby (Petric) to leave Birmingham for several years.

On several occasions, Petric shared with me how afraid he was to do what he chose to do, exposing his uncle for his part in the Sixteenth Street Baptist Church bombing and the many other atrocities he committed. However, my friend did not let fear stop him from standing up courageously to do the right thing by refusing to participate in or perpetuate a system he knew was, and is, wrong.

White supremacist ideology and White privilege cannot remain alive in a world that accepts Jesus. Remaining passive in a culture of silence keeps these ideologies alive. Acknowledging we are individuals who are part of God's big human family is vital to loving our neighbor as ourselves. Yes, we are different in many ways. But we are vastly more alike in that each of us is born with genetic characteristics over which we have no control.

I present as wholly White. I did not choose my skin color. You may be Black or Brown. You did not choose the color of your skin, either.

I am gay. I did not choose to be gay. Maybe you are, too. Maybe you are straight. Regardless, you did not choose your sexual orientation, either.

I was born in the United States to an unwed teenage mother. I did not choose my mother or my birth country. You may have

We Are Part of God's Big Family

been born in similar circumstances or in a different country. You did not choose that, either.

I was adopted. Maybe you were too.

I was raised in the Christian church. You may have been raised Jewish, Muslim, Buddhist, Hindu, another religion, or atheist.

We are different. Yet we are alike in our desire to love and be loved. We want to live safe from injustice, persecution, corruption, and judgment. We want to raise our children in a respectful, unpolluted, and peaceful world.

As a species that has been to the moon, cured diseases, built cities, and sent telescopes into deep space, we are certainly capable of moving ourselves forward to achieve ethnic and religious harmony. To create harmony, we need to admit the personal and collective hurt we have to heal is our ego's fear of difference, which fuels a lack of love and respect for ourselves and other people.

I know this sounds like a simple, pat answer. However, we know this is the right answer, as loving our neighbor as ourselves is the solution the soul named Jesus began teaching us millennia ago.

Isn't it time we listen, learn, and grow?

No child enters the world as a harbinger of fear, hate, prejudice, and disrespect. These responses are taught and learned. Love, acceptance, and respect are also taught and learned. That means we can choose to lead with our hearts and souls and be people who value compassion and integrity. Wouldn't Jesus want us to appreciate that being an honorable person of integrity and empathy is the greatest accomplishment we can achieve in life?

Some people think we should pray for God to take care of what is wrong with society and our world. Prayer is excellent, as long as we realize God is waiting for *us* to fix what is wrong—

CHAPTER 13

to fix the issues we created. You and I have not personally created everything negative in society, of course, but as part of our human family, we collectively allow global negatives such as greed, environmental destruction, and discrimination to exist.

Regardless what negatives we are challenged to face, first we have to admit there is no superhero coming to our rescue. God gave each of us the strength and willpower to change our lives, relationships, and world for the better. So God is waiting for each of us to step up and take the positive actions necessary every day to be the inclusive, peaceful, and loving change we want to see.

This raises two critical questions:

How can we rationalize waiting for a savior to rescue us when we need to be our own saviors by addressing our challenges head-on?
And unless we are dedicated to being people of integrity and empathy, how can we possibly work to right our wrongs?

The solution to the problems we face is really very simple: we cultivate a very clear sense of good and evil.

Good = honest, kind, responsible, inclusive, humble, forgiving, peaceful, respectful, nonviolent, ethical, and thoughtful (to name a few traits).

Evil = dishonest, cruel, irresponsible, divisive, arrogant, blaming, disrespectful, violent, corrupt, and thoughtless (to name a few traits).

There is no ambiguity between good and evil. The side on which we stand is clearly evident through the words we speak, the beliefs and attitudes we hold, and the behaviors we display. As Jesus says in Matthew 7: "You will know them by their fruits. Are grapes gathered from thorns or figs from thistles? In the same way, every good tree bears good fruit, but the bad tree bears bad

We Are Part of God's Big Family

fruit. A good tree cannot bear bad fruit, nor can a bad tree bear good fruit. Every tree that does not bear good fruit will be cut down and thrown into the fire. Thus you will know them by their fruits" (7:16–20).

To genuinely honor Jesus, it is essential for the church to lead the way in teaching the importance of walking in the footsteps of Jesus. The church has a duty to shape messages based on how respect for ourselves and others is reflected in our consistent dedication to living in integrity and empathy.

A "holier-than-thou" theology will never make us "chosen" in God's eyes.

I asked my Christian minister friend, Tim, why some Christians continue to see it as their duty to renounce and persecute other religions. He replied in a March 11, 2018, email:

> In spite of the influx of immigrants into the United States from across South America, Europe, Africa and beyond, representing a dynamic religious diversity, our citizens still consider us a Christian nation. And yet, most large American cities don't just have Protestant and Catholic churches everywhere, but now, Muslim mosques, Hindu and Buddhist temples, New Age meditation centers, Indian ashrams, Churches of Freethought (atheist), and more. . . .
>
> This is partially why so many Christians don't recognize other religions as valid, spiritual, God inspired, or capable of giving them eternal life through the belief there is only eternal salvation in Jesus Christ. Many of our Christian churches remain locked in their own traditions, convinced what they believe is the most authentic truth about God and salvation. If I am so fearful that someone else's faith or religious beliefs might somehow invalidate or transcend my own if I were to

CHAPTER 13

seriously consider them, then it is not surprising I remain frozen in my faith system.

Instead of opening our hearts and minds to the possibility God comes to us in a variety of ways, across many paths of belief and experience, we too often ignore and dismiss other faith systems and miss out on opportunities to experience God in new and profound ways. We fail to grow in the love Jesus invited us to share with him.

When Christians take responsibility and apologize for all the injustices we commit against one another, we will finally be honoring the sacrifice of Jesus.

Christians have the opportunity to love as Jesus did and take the lead in being an example of all that is good in Jesus's teachings of inclusion and empathy. Doing so requires the church to clean up the evil that is allowed to exist within the religion created in Christ's name, no matter how that wickedness manifests. To love Jesus, we cannot passively sit on the sidelines waiting for someone else to go first. We must go first and get creative by accepting the wisdom of Albert Einstein (and this one he really did say): "A new type of thinking is essential if mankind is to survive and move toward higher levels."[62]

Those of us who love Jesus are to bring a higher awareness to each harmful and unjust situation we face. To end mistreatment of one another, we need to do what Christ would do and go first, setting the example of treating all people as we want to be treated.

We practice the Golden Rule by associating with people of different skin colors, sexual orientations, and socioeconomic groups. We expose ourselves and our children to different cultures, customs, and religions.

We Are Part of God's Big Family

When we embrace all members of our human family, we will learn to have compassion for one another's challenges. We will listen to one another in order to understand, not just to respond. We will get to know one another in order to relate in intelligent and informed ways. We will appreciate our differences as well as our sameness.

Each of us is a member of the human race. We must no longer elevate ourselves, fear difference, or devalue others. We must focus on living with integrity by valuing compassion, responsibility, and kindness. We have to teach these values to our children as important skills they need to create a peaceful, courteous, and successful life. Consequently, Jesus would ask each Christian, and follower of any religion, to remember this: God looks past our outer human shell to determine the quality of our heart.

God desires we do the same by leading with our souls to see ourselves in all people. God wants us to respect the beautiful tapestry of humankind so we can create the world Jesus envisioned. To do so, we must intentionally keep our hearts open.

14

To Heal, We Must Feel

When I was eleven years old, I was hit in the head with a baseball bat. It was an accident. I was playing baseball with a few kids from the neighborhood in the backyard of our home on Locust Street in Victoria, Texas. I was catching. I did not think my playmate would swing at the badly pitched ball, so I moved forward. She did swing—and hit me on my left temple with the thick part of the bat.

I screamed. My skull pounded for hours, and my vision was blurry. I was sick to my stomach and thought I would faint. Although I was not taken to the doctor, I am certain I suffered a concussion. I know for sure the violent blow injured my neck and jaw, as decades later I still have discomfort.

This painful childhood experience taught me some valuable lessons. For example, I learned to avoid making assumptions about people or circumstances. I also learned no one gets right back up from being hit in the head, as we see them do in violent video games, on television, or in the movies. A shock to our physical system from a traumatic injury knocks us to our knees. Our body's spontaneous reaction is uncontrollable; we cannot help but cry, shout out, or faint. Once the initial intensity of physical

To Heal, We Must Feel

pain quiets down, the aches in our body and in our emotions can serve to remind us that everyone, and all life, feels.

To honor Jesus and truly heal the ills of society, don't we have to feel what other people feel? And if we want to genuinely feel the suffering of other people, isn't the first step to acknowledge our own suffering?

Feeling for others requires we first feel for ourselves. You can imagine the initial agony of being hit in the head with a baseball bat. Still, no matter how badly our bodies are damaged, terrible temporary physical pain pales in comparison to lasting emotional pain. The profound emotional wounding I experienced growing up gay and abused under judgmental, fearful, and controlling religious dogma hurt worse and did far more damage. For too many years, I was unable to productively express the deep misery, unworthiness, and loneliness I experienced. I felt isolated and undeserving of healthy, loving connections with people. I did not want to be seen. With no support and no one with whom I could share my pain, the anguish, isolation, and social stigma against expressing feelings forced me to keep my emotions bottled up tight. However, the unexpressed hurt I worked so hard to ignore was always there simmering, then bubbling, then inevitably boiling over.

At the age of eighteen, when the top blew, I raged and became self-destructive and abusive toward other people. I was arrogant, sarcastic, and condescending, venting and trying unsuccessfully to deal with the seething indignation I harbored at being unfairly judged. I was angry with God for making me gay and then abandoning me. I hated being bullied by mean and insecure people. I was mad about having been sexually abused. I was furious with men for attempting to control and suppress women in general. I was upset with myself for being different and, therefore, in my mind, unworthy. And I was distressed at not having anyone with whom to

CHAPTER 14

share my pain and confusion. I could not even share it with God, since it was made clear to me God hated me for being gay.

Even if I had had someone to share with, most likely I would not have. I was raised under the command "If you don't have anything nice to say, don't say anything at all." Society taught me people who talked about their feelings or confronted different perspectives or beliefs were pushy and lacked manners. That sounded a lot like the command I received not to challenge the Bible because I would be blasphemous for going against God.

Why do we often silence someone from speaking their truth? Why do we invalidate the experiences of those who share their feelings? What do we have to fear from that? Wouldn't Jesus want those who love him to listen to and learn from the stories of those who are hurting?

My parents were raised with the social edict that it was inappropriate to express feelings; therefore, when I was a child and young adult, if I violated the preferred behavior of being polite rather than being honest, I was punished. Even now, when conversations with my parents get tense, their training prompts them to quickly change the topic or tell me I am too emotional.

That is hardly healthy. Embracing our emotions is part of loving ourselves. But instead of being shown how to deal with the wide range of our emotions in constructive ways, we are taught to invalidate our feelings. We are often mocked by family and peers for feeling what we do. We may be told we are unworthy of Jesus's or God's love or not good enough to walk in the footsteps of Jesus. We might be warned we are going to hell.

Generations of us have been taught to avoid conflict and authenticity in favor of conforming. Yet being forced to stuff our feelings down distances us from our hearts. Without the ability to establish emotional intimacy through responsibly expressing

To Heal, We Must Feel

what we think and feel, we don't know how to positively deal with tension or differences in our relationships. As a result, many of us are afraid of productive disagreement.

Many of us were told it is not okay for us to feel bad either because it makes other people uncomfortable or because Christians are supposed to always be joyful. The truth is, when we are treated badly or suffer abuse, we will feel bad. That's not only the natural response; it's the correct one. We cannot escape what we feel, especially when the mistreatment, neglect, and invalidation of our emotions continue.

Jesus would say it is okay to feel bad at times. He would also encourage us to look at why we feel the way we do, with the goal of embracing our emotions in order to heal.

If we don't validate our distress, how can we love ourselves?
Isn't it unhealthy to believe we can love if we don't allow ourselves to express our true feelings?
Would Jesus want us to avoid acting abusively toward ourselves as well as other people?

Self-abusive behavior makes us think it is okay to abuse other people. I am certain Jesus knows we are being phony each time we attempt to portray ourselves as spiritually healthy yet participate in self-abusive habits or abuse other people. We have to remember loving Jesus is a full-time job, one of striving daily to become proficient in walking in his emotionally healthy footsteps. Proficiency comes from becoming aware of what we need to change within ourselves so we transform negative, hurtful behavior into positive and loving conduct.

Doesn't the church have the obligation to encourage and support our emotional health?

CHAPTER 14

But the church seems to be confused about the vital role it plays in helping to create emotionally healthy people. By not emphasizing emotional health, by not helping to build our self-esteem, inner worth, and connection to and respect for one another, the church is contributing to the development of emotionally dysfunctional adults and children.

Our lack of empathy is clear in a variety of abusive behaviors we inflict on ourselves. In futile attempts to escape feeling our buried pain, we overeat or undereat. We drink too much or abuse dangerously addictive drugs of all kinds. We cut ourselves or may otherwise self-harm. We dismiss speed limits, run stop signs, ignore traffic signals, or text and drive, justifying that convenience is more important than safety.

Refusing to let ourselves genuinely express what we feel keeps us disconnected from our hearts. Without being connected to our emotions, we blame other people for our negative behaviors rather than assume responsibility for our actions. We project our shortcomings onto others rather than look to ourselves for the solution to our stress and unhappiness. We live in our heads, constantly justifying or rationalizing away personal struggles instead of giving them much-needed attention. We overwork, have affairs, believe conspiracy theories, and remain tied to technology because these outlets allow us to feel something, even if it's not the actual emotions we have numbed. Wouldn't Jesus want us to stay connected to our feelings in order to find fulfillment?

God designed us to feel our way through life. Without embracing our emotions, our relationships are often superficial. We keep ourselves so busy we don't have time to feel. Without expressing what we feel in healthy ways, we have no clue how to support other people in expressing healthy emotion, either.

When we cannot safely express our feelings, voice our needs, or present our viewpoints, we often turn our frustration inward.

To Heal, We Must Feel

We may harbor resentment, anger, and unworthiness. These emotions fester and can cause us to explode, often on those who are closest to us, like a spouse or partner or child. Or we shut down and lose our ability to speak up about anything.

Being silenced, abused, or discounted causes us to lose confidence in ourselves. Without the self-confidence to speak up, we don't challenge the abusive behavior of other people. We don't admit our own self-abuse. We don't stand up for ourselves. We bury our emotions and feel invalidated and unworthy. We become codependent or passive-aggressive in our relationships. We don't ask for what we want. We become self-centered and irresponsibly inflict our suffering on those we say we love. Isn't admitting we're hurting ourselves or other people a positive first step toward healing?

While growing up, one of my friends, Peter, was used as a punching bag by his alcoholic father. He was the frequent target of his father's misplaced rage, disappointment, and feelings of inadequacy. Yet Peter grew up to become a loving, peaceful, and thoughtful father. Long ago he made the deliberate choice not to be like his own father. He broke the cycle of abuse by assuming responsibility for dealing with his emotional wounds. Peter did not want to take his abuse out on himself, other people, or other living things.

Peter realized his father did not know to look inside himself to address whatever abuse he had endured in his own past that caused him to drown his emotional pain with alcohol and lash out at his family. My friend's father did not question his actions. But my friend knows we are emotional beings who need to look within and heal the holes in our heart so we don't let our pain dictate how we treat other adults or children and animals. One of the most loving things for parents to do is address the holes within their hearts so they don't pass their wounding on to their children.

CHAPTER 14

For many years, I never saw my father express any emotion other than anger. He grew up in a society where "real" men did not cry or talk about their feelings. He knew if a man or boy expressed healthy emotion through crying or identified his feelings through productive sharing, he would be labeled by his peers, and even by many women, as a "momma's boy," "faggot," or "crybaby." On the other hand, if my father got angry, it seemed permissible, and even expected, that he be free to release his pent-up rage, no matter how his words and actions negatively affected those around him.

"You're too emotional," he once said coldly, as tears streamed down my face during the nature documentaries he watched that included horrific scenes of baby harp seals being beaten to death and close-up, slow-motion images of prairie dogs being blown to bits.

My father repeatedly slammed the broken closet door in my bedroom. One day, when Dad and I were playing catch outside, he spotted a hole in my T-shirt and ripped it off. I once saw him kick our little dog, Penny. Our other dog, Caesar, was terrified during thunderstorms. The big golden lab threw himself against the garage door, trying to get in, or cowered in his doghouse and made pitiful sounds. It broke my heart to see him afraid. I understood how it felt to be frightened, with nowhere to hide and no one to offer comfort. I was powerless to offer help to the miserable dog. My father threatened the belt if I let Caesar into the garage or even went outside to be with him.

My father stormed through life not seeming to give a damn about the feelings of other living things. His temper tantrums, sarcastic remarks, and occasional drunken hecklings during my youth softball games further confirmed he was often a cold, callous, and uncaring man.

To Heal, We Must Feel

Then one beautiful, crisp autumn day, that changed.

He was hunting and knew he had fatally wounded a deer, but he could not find it. It went against his values to leave the deer, so he searched for hours without success. At the end of the day he was so exhausted and upset, he sat down on a log, buried his head in his hands, and sobbed, maybe for the first time—or at least the first time in many, many years.

I feel privileged because later in life, my dad began to share with me some of the emotional and physical abuse he had experienced. For the first five years of his life, his mother, because of physical limitations, could not pick him up. Whether purposefully or unconsciously, her inability to consistently hold my dad caused him to feel ignored and unwanted. My father was an only child whose mother seemed to abandon him. He did not receive the crucial love, attention, and touch necessary for him to be able to respond to his own emotional needs or those of his family, leaving him distant, unfeeling, and often unkind.

Growing up, my dad was disciplined by those who believed in the adage "Spare the rod and spoil the child." He was invalidated by those who adhered to the maxim "Children are to be seen and not heard." Following these cruel ideas about child-rearing, some family members treated him appallingly. They criticized, belittled, and humiliated him. When he was a teenager he was staying with a relative. After attending an event in town, he had to walk several miles on foot back to the house of the relative, who had imposed a curfew on him. The relative locked him out of the house because he was five minutes late.

Puritanical cruelty is not, and never was, Christlike. Like me, my father was raised with his own strict religious judgment and suffered under the hellfire-and-damnation dogma of his church experiences. Christian ministers and churchgoers in his

CHAPTER 14

family placed harsh punishments and unrealistic expectations on him.

My dad underwent great emotional and physical pain, much of it inflicted by those who were supposed to care for him and protect him. The same people who said they loved Jesus and God were anything but loving. He was heartlessly taught to shut off emotion.

No matter how much we suffered, those in authority made it clear to both my father and me that we were to take it. We were instructed to basically lie and say all was well instead of honestly acknowledging our pain and sharing it with one another.

Being gentle with ourselves and all life is one of the strongest things we do. Children learn acceptable or unacceptable behavior from their parents, but how can parents wrap their arms around their children while clinging to the heavy baggage of their own emotional wounding? Why do we often say "I'm sorry" when we cry or get choked up, as if we need to apologize for our emotions? We learn to honor the emotions of other people through the process of honoring our emotions.

How can we ignore our inner pain and expect to have wholesome relationships or live a life of peace, self-respect, and genuine love? Part of loving ourselves is facing the wounding we experience in childhood.

We cannot love ourselves and other people unless our hearts are free of suffering to make room for compassion and empathy. It is time for the church to focus intently on honoring Jesus's suffering by helping to boost our self-esteem rather than helping to perpetuate our unworthiness and shame.

Remember way back in chapter 2 when I mentioned watching that sad-looking man distribute fear-based religious tracts? The hellfire-and-damnation pamphlet left on my doorstep that day showed me that, still, too many who say they love Jesus are

To Heal, We Must Feel

caught up in punishing themselves and others rather than learning how to love themselves so they can love others. We are in an epidemic of unworthy feelings. This is evident because we would not treat ourselves and other people badly if we were encouraged by the church, our families, and society to feel and express healthy emotion.

Regardless of gender, we are specifically designed to feel our way through life. Some people may argue women are better at expressing their feelings than men. I believe this is true not because we are so different but because there is greater social stigma attached to men expressing emotion. To move past this negative social dynamic, both men and women need to remember, Jesus readily expressed his feelings.

Jesus wept. He loved. He hurt.

Jesus was a man who had to be intimately in touch with his emotions in order to love the way he did. Yet for me, and maybe for you also, the importance of embracing and freely sharing emotion in healthy ways was neither emphasized nor modeled by the Christian church. Therefore, the church owes it to a feeling Jesus to step up and lead discussions about how our emotional health is vital to our spiritual health, because we need much more than prayer for one another.

For me, my dad, and anyone who has been bullied and abused, it is necessary to positively deal with the residual wounding that manifests as emotional distance and irresponsible behavior. When our egotistical or fear-based actions result in harming ourselves and other people, we need to look at ourselves honestly. To do so, we need to be okay with seeking help.

An effective way to heal is to talk about our pain with a trusted friend, spouse, minister, or counselor—someone who offers a safe space to release negative emotion. Someone like my friend

CHAPTER 14

Byll, who sat with me, supportive and nonjudgmental, as I waded through years of traumatic events. He did not tell me what I needed to do. He simply listened, wanting to understand, and offered support, which allowed me to release much of what was continuing to cause me to suffer.

Talking about our feelings and experiences and expressing our needs are vital to creating emotionally intimate relationships, including the relationship we have with ourselves and Jesus. True intimacy is baring ourselves to another who holds our hearts safe.

It takes enormous courage and willpower to speak about mistreatment we experience or witness. It takes determination to overcome the fear of being ridiculed, not taken seriously, or punished for speaking up. However, one of the most productive things we can do is acknowledge what we feel—anger, sadness, unworthiness, fear, or shame—by talking about the pain and memories, which allows us to find our voice again. Wouldn't Jesus tell us asking for help is a sign not of weakness but of strength?

I also consulted several counselors in my process of letting go of a painful past. Each professional counselor I saw offered a key to building my self-esteem so I could move on. That is why I know one of the most loving actions we take is that of confiding in people who can help us name what we feel, people who encourage us to acknowledge each emotion we experience.

In addition to trusted people with whom to share, we may need bodywork help to release the physical pain stored in our bodies we may not even be aware of.

When I was very young, my mother cut her wrist when a big ceramic pickle vat fell off the counter and shattered on the floor. I was outside and heard her scream for me. I raced inside. She told me to run and get a neighbor. I was so scared and ran as fast as I could. On the way, I tripped, fell, scraped my knee, and twisted

To Heal, We Must Feel

my ankle. I managed to limp the rest of the way and got the neighbor, and my mom was taken to the hospital for stitches.

I don't remember ever thinking about my ankle after that day. It seemed to heal without giving me much trouble. Many years later, I was having Rolfing bodywork done—a type of therapy that manipulates the fasciae in our body that connect all our bones, muscles, ligaments, and tendons. When the therapist got to my ankle, without warning I began to cry. Yes, there was a little pain, but the tears were caused by the flood of memories of my mother and those events. It is so interesting how my body kept the memories, and after so many years, they surfaced.

Our bodies are amazing storehouses of information. Sometimes we need help from a therapist to release an emotional trauma or uncomfortable experience we may have forgotten but our body still remembers. This embodiment of emotional trauma is something the Inipi ceremony also helped me confront. The physical discomfort was intense and cleansing. Enduring the heat and the flood of painful memories allowed me to gain a deeper appreciation for how strong we are, physically and mentally, to deal with and overcome the challenges we face in life.

> *Wouldn't Jesus remind us we have the strength to release the resentment and suffering we hold onto about anything hurtful we experience in life?*
> *Don't we honor Jesus's suffering by healing our own?*
> *Don't healed people help other people heal because their increased self-compassion and respect in turn model empathy and respect for others?*

Life is filled with challenges. We are bombarded by the highs and lows of emotion. We need to accept that healthy emotional

CHAPTER 14

release is part of daily living. When we validate and honor our emotions and express them in healthy ways, we can support other people in expressing their emotions in healthy ways, too.

I believe we are all crying out for healing in one way or another. When we commit ourselves to a healthy path in pursuit of this goal—of healing our wounding or getting control over an addiction—we do whatever it takes to accomplish the goal. We want to heal as badly as a drowning person wants air. We realize healing is not something we can do casually on weekends or in just one hour a week with a counselor. We recognize healing is a radical lifestyle change. Living healed becomes our reason for being, our moment-by-moment priority.

It takes intentional effort to arrive at the place of being ready to be free of past emotional trauma. I believe to honor the sacrifice of Jesus, it is essential for the church to help lead the way in working to end all shame around expressing healthy emotions. We teach our young girls and boys positive ways to name their emotions and express their feelings. We encourage one another to feel what we feel. We nurture self-worth and respect in one another. We share life's highs and lows with people we trust to hold our hearts safe. We allow ourselves to be seen by other people—our strengths and weaknesses.

When we embrace our emotions and encourage other people to do the same, we will learn to love one another as Jesus loved.

15

Love One Another as Jesus Loved

Think about this with me for a moment: *Love is the action of making the invisible care and affection we have for ourselves and other people visible, through positive action.*

I believe Jesus would say this is exactly how we can define love. And patience. And compassion, respect, and more—our integrity on display.

Yet no matter how simple and logical this idea of "love" seems, it took a chance meeting with a stranger for me to really understand that love is, indeed, the positive behaviors of our integrity in action. And in hindsight, I realize this person was not really a stranger at all but a messenger of God who appeared in my life quite deliberately—just in an unexpected disguise.

It was in the alcove of a storefront, close to the corner of Fairfax and Wilshire in Los Angeles, California, where I sobbed in this homeless man's arms. I did not know the man. Most likely I will not see him again. But I will not forget the moment our hearts touched in the intimate dance of raw truth: he lives on the street, and I, in a warm apartment.

Our exchange began when I complimented his dog. He smiled very proudly and said, "Yeah, she's great. I've got her back and she's got mine."

CHAPTER 15

As he spoke, he gently petted the dog. I reached into my wallet and took out all the money I had and handed it to him.

He hesitantly took it. As our hands touched, my tears began. The man reached out, wrapped me in his arms, and said, "It is okay. We're okay out here. Thank you for caring."

As I turned to leave, he said, "I love you."

I looked him in the eyes and said, "I love you, too."

Until then I had never said "I love you" to a complete stranger, someone I had just met and with whom I had exchanged only a few brief moments of conversation. However, when he spoke love to me and I spontaneously responded "I love you, too," I meant it from the bottom of my heart. There was no judgment. My soul was simply wide open, and pure, honest caring came pouring out not because I was moved by my own generosity but because Jesus had spoken clearly in that moment.

I saw that man and his dog and could have passed them by. But I heard Jesus within my heart say, *See him, and tell him he is seen!*

My choice to listen to and act upon Jesus's direction opened me to a lesson I was able to learn only with the willingness to experience the sincerity of our exchange. Holding the man and allowing him to hold me birthed a deep and profound understanding of what it means to be vulnerable to caring, without expectations or conditions. The kind of openness we want to experience. The depth of intimacy we long for. The wonder of being connected to the unconditional love of Jesus in ourselves and in another human being.

Isn't that the goal of Christianity, after all—to teach us to love one another as Jesus loved?

When I was young, my mother said, "We never know if someone we meet may be one of God's angels" (see Hebrews 13:2). My sweet unhoused man was an angel. He was God's messenger of

Love One Another as Jesus Loved

wisdom who taught me love is more than caring and affection for those closest to us.

Each of us experiences countless transformational moments in life—occasions when we are given the opportunity to advance the ability we have, as souls, to let unconditional love move through us without allowing fear, judgment, or expectation to stop us.

Certainly the close relationships we have are the most important part of life. We have deep fondness for and personal attachments to some people and pets. They are special to us and add to our lives. We definitely would miss them if they were no longer around.

Yet no matter how deeply we care for our family and friends, every exchange we have with another human being, animal, and the natural world is an opportunity to fully feel our magnificent heart connection to *all* that is alive. Because *love is who we are, when we allow ourselves to be it.*

Jesus lived as love. To love him, we must do the same. The caring and affection he had for the world flowed organically through him and was visible as his honorable behavior. Consequently, for us, love is also the caring and affection we have for ourselves, other people, and all life that is displayed as our honorable behavior in action.

Jesus was—and is—the embodiment of love. Therefore, to love Jesus, aren't we to be ambassadors of love too?

Jesus was patient, kind, and respectful. He forgave people and was responsible for himself. He was cooperative, attentive, and peaceful. The honorable behaviors of love Jesus displayed—consistently treating people as he wanted to be treated—originated from the soul he was. Therefore, his soul and ours are home to integrity, which we feel and express as love. When we love as Jesus did, we cause honorable integrity to move through us.

CHAPTER 15

But in order to let our love flow, without judgment or conditions, we have to overrule the part of us (ego) that does not care whether we behave from our soul's integrity or not.

In the exchange I had with the homeless man, I could have ignored the "Jesus calling" I heard. In fact, if I had listened to my ego, I would have kept on walking. The man was dirty and smelled bad. Maybe he would hurt or rob me. He should get a job. The dog might have had fleas. There were numerous fear-based excuses for why I should not stop.

Instead of giving in to judgmental excuses, though, I chose to follow Jesus's direction and act from the nonjudgmental and unconditional acceptance of my heart. My heart did not care about the man's tattered clothing, dirt, or body odor; it led me to hold him in my arms without scorn. My soul cared only about his kind spirit. In return, his soul accepted and returned my loving-kindness.

Although I was raised under the continual threat of hellfire and damnation, I don't believe in a flesh-and-blood, hell-based Satan figure who desires to steal my soul or who controls my behavior. Yet there is a real draw to our uncaring and judgmental side—the idea that there is a literal evil entity steering our steps as it plans to derail our path to salvation. It makes us believe we are better than those poor souls who are in the devil's clutches. It shifts the blame for our bad decisions from our own egos to some outside force. The temptation to submit to fearful and controlling ego rather than follow the loving prompts of the very soul we are is a challenge you and I experience countless times every day. We will face these moment-by-moment, ego-versus-soul choices as long as we live.

In my experiences with the rude man in the coffee shop and the young Christian people on the elevator, my ego wanted me to blast

Love One Another as Jesus Loved

them. However, ego is not the part of us that has integrity. Ego has no moral and responsible rudder to steer us in the direction of what Jesus would do. When the unhealthy part of us, lacking the respect and restraint of integrity, rears its ugly head, we want to ego box with people. Or we want to control or change them. It is at those times that we need to question whether our thoughts, words, attitudes, and beliefs are aligned with Jesus-like love.

As you know, I quietly (and toxically) held onto the biggest secret of my life until it almost killed me. To save my life, I was forced to break the silence that was keeping me trapped in isolation and shame, and I told my parents the truth about my being gay. I could not live a lie, which is exactly what my fearful ego wanted me to do.

Upon hearing the news, their first thought was that I had to change to become heterosexual. Many people are led to believe converting, changing, and controlling other people is how we love them, that it is for their own good. *Love does not attempt to change or control others.*

It was ego that wanted me to change into my parents' and society's idea of normal. Love knows I did not need to be changed. God made me the way I am. What I needed was their support (love) to help me learn how to navigate a world where people like me are bullied, persecuted, and continuously threatened with spending eternity in hell.

When we stop and think, we realize that relationships where ego is allowed to enter into the mix result in self-control, caring, logic, and respect going out the window. Ego wants what it wants, when it wants it. Ego is all about domination. The problem with control is it is not love.

So how do we overcome our ego in order to reliably lead with our heart's integrity?

CHAPTER 15

Although it may seem counterintuitive, the way we manage our ego so we can love other people as Jesus wants us to is by first loving ourselves. I know this concept is probably the opposite of what you were taught. If you are like me, you were told loving yourself first is selfish. But loving ourselves first is not selfish; *it is responsible.*

Think about it.

Many of us were taught to believe it is our duty to love someone else before we love ourselves. I was taught to care for Jesus and God and other people before myself. Consequently, I spent much of my life attempting to do so, and I failed miserably.

We all fail at this.

Why?

We are not taught what loving ourselves really feels like—to consistently treat ourselves with respect and care. Only then can we give the feelings of love to others because we now understand it.

For example, when we are patient with ourselves first, we will know what patience feels like. When we experience the serenity of patience, we can give others the feeling of peacefulness by being patient with them. Likewise, when we are compassionate with ourselves first, we know the feeling of empathy and can genuinely give this value of love to someone. When we forgive ourselves for our mistakes, we feel the freedom that comes from being responsible for our actions and for making amends to those we harm. Self-love in the form of self-forgiveness fills us with the love required to forgive the mistakes of others.

Every time we give the behaviors of love to ourselves first, we are filled with the feeling of loving. We can then express those feelings of love to others. Also, when we give love's behaviors to ourselves first, should life present occasions when the depth of our self-love (integrity in action) is truly put to a test, we can rise to the challenge.

We must love ourselves first to love others well. Let me explain what I mean.

A man I know, Gerome, was walking to work early in the morning when he smelled something burning, then spotted smoke coming from beneath the door of a house in his neighborhood. He knew an old man lived alone in the home. Gerome called 9-1-1 for the fire department while he banged loudly on the front door. When there was no response, he grabbed a chair from the front porch, pushed it through a window, and went into the smoke-filled house. Staying low to the ground, he crawled around until he found the old man in bed. He carried him out the front door and laid him on the grass. A few minutes later, the fire department and medical response people arrived and took over. The old man pulled through, though his faulty space heater had almost cost him his home *and* his life.

Gerome received an award from the city for his heroic act. He also got attention from the media and other organizations for his kind and brave actions. The old man and his family expressed their gratitude with a special dinner for him.

My friend did not think what he did was special. He believed anyone would have done the same in his position. Yet not everyone would have risked their life to save another the way Gerome did. That makes him a true hero, because while he was in the right place at the right time, he *intentionally chose to be love in action.*

Gerome chose to love himself first by remaining true to his commitment to be of help to those in need. Even though it put his own life in danger, he knew in his heart he would not have been able to love or respect himself if he had chosen to simply walk away that day. My friend learned that loving ourselves first

CHAPTER 15

sometimes demands a willingness to risk everything in order to stay in line with what makes our souls whole and gives meaning to our lives: being people of integrity. We must first have love within in order to be able to give love to others. And treating ourselves with the values of love first is vital because only self-love inspires us to overrule ego.

Courage is inspired by loving ourselves first, which enables us to lead with the positive character values that display our integrity. It does not take courage to act from ego. For example, have you lied and watched anxiously as the lie began to weave a web of deceit?

I have. More than once. I now know how important it is to be honest in order to create fulfilling relationships and a peaceful life. However, the only way I could learn the dangers of allowing ego to direct my behavior was by realizing that each time I lied, I was actually being a coward. I was not brave enough to remain aligned with my integrity and tell the truth regardless of the consequences. I excused lying as a good way to cover up something I did or I knew was wrong. Or I lied in a misguided attempt to make myself look more important than I was or so I would not have to be honest when someone asked my opinion about them.

I rationalized lying as being harmless.

No one would find out, right?

The truth is, truth always comes out, eventually and assuredly, shining a bright spotlight on our character (or lack thereof).

By lying, no matter what justification we create to defend our dishonesty, we have knowingly betrayed ourselves and other people. Each time we choose to lie, we feel the negative impact. We instantly become caught in a sticky web that grows as one lie weaves two more. Two weave four. Four weave sixteen, and on and on until we are completely stuck in our trap of dishonesty.

Love knows doing the right thing is always the right thing to do. No matter how hard it is to stay aligned with the integrity of soul

Love One Another as Jesus Loved

and tell the truth, being honest with ourselves and other people is an act of personal power and self-respect. Sure, it can be quite challenging to always tell the truth. The temptation to avoid embarrassment or punishment, or to defend our fragile pride (ego), is often hard to resist, and rather than remain honorable, we lie. However, honesty is vital to establishing trust.

God tells us the right thing to do within the quiet prompts of our heart. Aren't we the ones with power to listen and obey or to ignore?

Truthfulness is the foundation of all successful relationships, including the one we have with ourselves. Only by being honest rather than following unethical ego can we avoid becoming trapped in the web of hell created by dishonesty. Therefore, loving ourselves is having the courage to be completely truthful.

Love is a choice we make to do the right thing. That motivation originates in our soul's integrity.

Doesn't it make sense for us to give the behaviors of love's integrity to ourselves first before we can give them to other people? When we are honest with ourselves, we will be honest with others. Being kind to ourselves teaches us how to be kind to other people and all life. Supporting ourselves shows us how to support others. Respecting ourselves fills us with the empathy required to respect other people. Caring for ourselves allows us to know what it feels like to be cared for. When we fill ourselves with unconditional and responsible love, we can give honest love.

It is through loving ourselves that we become emotionally invested in the outcome so we make ourselves take the actions necessary to realize any goal. *Love motivates us to grow into better versions of ourselves.*

A young woman I know graduated from college with honors. While this achievement is not rare, for her to do so was an exceptional accomplishment. For many years, she attempted to battle her inner demons by abusing crystal meth. She lived on

CHAPTER 15

the street, stole from her parents, traded sex for drugs, was in and out of countless treatment programs, and watched friends die.

One day she woke up to the way she was behaving by accepting that she had to love and respect herself in order to put an end to a life of suffering. The people who cared for her were not able to do this for her. Only by caring for and valuing herself did she find the motivation and determination to do what it took to turn her life around.

The process of inner deliberation, with the intention of making positive change, awakens us to our irresponsible and self-abusive actions—a process that takes deep self-care and affection.

Each of us has to self-assess, with the goal of continuously transforming for the better. No matter how much we are cared for by other people, no one can do this work for us. Until we determine why we harbor resentment and anger, live in fear, believe ourselves unworthy, or abuse ourselves, we will not wake up to the truth that our behavior creates our lives, and we will not appreciate that how we think and feel about ourselves drives our behavior.

It takes conscious awareness to move through life caring about our thoughts, words, and actions. I know from experience stopping to ask ourselves how our behavior will feel—both to ourselves and to others—allows us to consult the integrity of our hearts.

When we appreciate that the caring we have for ourselves and other people is expressed as the positive behavior of our integrity, we will recognize ego-motivated treatment, which is not loving. When we care about the impact of our actions, chances are excellent we will choose what we do and say before we act, with the goal of creating the most responsible and loving outcome.

16

Love Has Excellent Vision

Most likely you are familiar with the phrase "Love is blind." This expression is first found in Chaucer's *The Merchant's Tale*, written between 1387 and 1400. The phrase did not come into common usage until William Shakespeare's tragedy *Romeo and Juliet*, in the scene in which Benvolio says to Mercutio, "Blind is his love, and best befits the dark" (act 2, scene 1). Mercutio responds that if love is blind, then it is not real love.

I agree: love (integrity in action) is not blind. Infatuation is blind, but our integrity is not. For us to treat ourselves and other people with the respect and caring Jesus desires we do, we need to be able to tell the difference between loving and nonloving behavior.

As the old expression goes, actions speak louder than words. A friend of mine has an unmarried adult daughter who became pregnant. My friend felt no stigma around her daughter's pregnancy; however, she had a problem with her daughter's boyfriend, who psychologically tormented, manipulated, and was disrespectful to her daughter. She also had difficulty with his mother, who defended her son's abuse.

The daughter excused the boyfriend, saying she loved him. She refused to listen to her mother or sister, both of whom asked

CHAPTER 16

her to see the man for what his repeated behavior revealed was the truth of his character. Their words fell on deaf ears because her infatuation with her boyfriend was blind. Infatuation sees what it wants to see.

With every fight, the daughter complained about how badly her boyfriend treated her. Each time, her mother and sister reasserted she had to end the relationship. But the young woman repeatedly refused to let the man go, believing her love was strong enough to change him. What she did not realize was that her love for *herself*—which would take the form of her integrity's self-respect, self-confidence, and worthiness—was not strong enough to say no and set healthy boundaries against his unhealthy abuse.

The daughter, like many of us, believed love endures all things. The truth is, our integrity cannot and should not withstand all things. While all relationships have challenges, affection expressed positively, as our soul's integrity, does not tolerate the dishonest or abusive actions of other people. No matter if someone is a family member or a close friend, we don't have to hang in there, allowing them to dump their anger, self-centeredness, and emotional unconsciousness onto us. How can our affection be genuine or lasting if it is based on a fantasy of what we hope someone or a relationship will be rather than the reality of what it is? It is one thing to see potential in someone, but a healthy relationship has to be built on something more than hopes and dreams for who they will be someday.

Tolerating abuse is not how to care for someone or ourselves. Our love may demand we rock the boat because for us to love as Jesus did, we need to know *turning the other cheek to abuse is a misconception about love that is wrong and unhealthy.*

It is one thing to let rude and self-centered (but not emotionally or physically abusive) behavior go, as I did with the young people on the elevator and the man in the coffee shop. But people who live an integrity-centered life are not submissive to abuse. We don't take it or allow it to continue.

Healthy relationships have healthy boundaries. To love one another as Jesus did, we accept that he set strong boundaries against nonloving behavior (look at the way he defended the woman who was threatened with stoning in John 8, for example), and he would encourage us to do so also.

Life is filled with situations in which loving as Jesus did requires us to set tough boundaries against nonloving behavior. To allow ourselves to be physically, emotionally, or psychologically abused in any relationship is not loving ourselves, nor is it loving those who are behaving badly. And if there are children involved, exposure to disrespect and abuse in a relationship causes them stress and teaches them unhealthy dynamics that are certainly not loving.

To love with the heart of Jesus and with the souls we are, we have to control our self-centered, arrogant, and critical sides. And we have to set boundaries with those who don't care to address their own ego-driven, hurtful behavior. Jesus took a firm stand against injustice and those who enabled the abuse of people.

By accepting personal responsibility for our behavior, we acknowledge there is no force outside us that directs our actions. You and I are completely responsible to God, Jesus, and ourselves for our behavior. We cannot go through life hurting ourselves and other people and disrespecting God's magnificent creations and expect to face no accountability for our actions simply by professing Jesus is our savior, by being baptized, or by attending church.

To save ourselves and others from the hell our destructive actions create, it is necessary for us to choose to walk in the footsteps of self-love and behave with Jesus-like integrity. Doing so often requires tough love for ourselves and other people because

CHAPTER 16

refusing to set a boundary against mistreatment is saying abusive behavior is acceptable. It is not.

Can anything be changed for the better without being faced head-on? No.

To love as Jesus did, we cannot be afraid of engaging in Jesus-like discord to condemn abuse in our personal, religious, political, and social relationships. We are brave, like Jesus, and choose authenticity over conforming to the socially acceptable culture of not wanting to be seen as a troublemaker. We remember Jesus was an agitator against those people who mistreated others. As John Lewis would say, "Never, ever be afraid to make some noise and get in good trouble, necessary trouble." Jesus would definitely get into good and necessary trouble as an activist against anyone or any organization that mistreats people. Therefore, you and I need to lead with the courage of Jesus. In our homes, churches, government, and society in general, we stand up to those who abuse because we must not turn the other cheek to mistreatment.

We accept that love is *not* blind. We refuse to be complicit in accepting harmful teachings as God's word or God's will. We are not afraid to stand alone against the crowd. We accept that Jesus would want us to care more about whom we entrust with positions of religious and political influence than we do about what other people think of us. I don't think it's a stretch to imagine Jesus would walk out of any religious service or political rally that promotes fear, exclusion, or disinformation or condones the persecution of fellow human beings.

Jesus would not care about what these types of people thought of him. He would not worry about being ridiculed over social media. He would not be concerned about being condemned by any false prophet or wannabe dictator who is addicted to the artificial attention they get from fame and power over people.

Love Has Excellent Vision

To love Jesus, we set Jesus-like boundaries. We turn off conspiracy theorists. We change the channel on religious evangelists and talk-show hosts who press falsehoods, political biases, and fear of others. We refuse to follow those who use social media as a platform to denigrate people or spread lies, abuse, and misinformation. We challenge the punditocracy, the powerful and influential political commentators. We appreciate that our news delivery model is based on algorithms designed to amplify division and encourage "doom scrolling," which results in our being overwhelmed with negative-reinforcing stories.

In the words of Robert Reich, American economist, lawyer, and retired professor at the Goldman School of Public Policy at the University of California, Berkeley, "The media (including social media) sells subscriptions and advertising with stories that generate anger and disappointment. The same goes for the views of pundits and commentators: Pessimists always appear wiser than optimists."[63]

Words have power because they create real outcomes.

Jesus would want us to use our words responsibly by accepting the consequences of what we say. That means Jesus would want us to separate ourselves from anyone, anywhere, who lies, divides, and creates chaos designed to instill fear and mistrust. And Jesus wants us to be courageous because when divisive-minded people are confronted on their un-Jesus-like behavior, they tend to turn on anyone who challenges them. But I think it's fair to assume Jesus would tell us, "Doing the right thing is always the right thing to do."

When we rise, as Jesus would, and walk out, tune out, delete, and confront those who lie, divide, and promote hatred and disinformation, we will not be able to prevent what they will say about us. The true characters of the people we thought we knew will be revealed. We will not be able to stop ego-motivated members of

CHAPTER 16

the religious congregations or political parties we leave from vilifying us. We will not prevent the negative fallout created by our family or friends who don't care to honestly examine exclusive and judgmental beliefs.

I know this isn't easy; I've been on the receiving end of slanderous behavior myself. I understand what a challenge it is to remain calm when there is gossip about you. Or when people you know are pressured to slander you. Or when there are manufactured stories about your personal business or your life.

The negative things said reveal much more about the person saying them than they do about the person who is being talked about. Remember, there is a long-established pattern in human history that when false prophets and those corrupted by power are exposed and challenged for who they are, they defensively cast suspicion and blame on other people.

I believe that to love Jesus, we courageously call out the rampant misuse of religious and political power by those who use the Bible as a weapon. We cannot be passive, silent, or uninformed about harmful policies simply because those policies don't affect us personally. We stand with Jesus on the side of people who are oppressed and marginalized. We courageously separate from those who divide and destroy, and we stand with Jesus and join with those who are inclusive, truthful, and supportive, who promote tangible ways to love one another as Jesus did.

No matter what situation we encounter in life, we have the choice to add to the problem or be part of the solution. While we cannot change anyone but ourselves, we can set necessary boundaries to maintain our integrity and devotion to what Jesus would do—and we can love as Jesus did.

So how did my friend deal with her daughter who wouldn't leave her abusive boyfriend?

Love Has Excellent Vision

Since the young woman would not look at the man for who he was and see his abusive treatment of her was not love, my friend knew her daughter did not care for herself. Without the self-respect necessary to honor herself, the daughter would have remained in this unhealthy dynamic.

In this case, my friend exercised a tough-love option. Since her daughter lived with her, she asked her daughter to leave her home. My friend knows love always seeks a positive outcome, even when in order to stop enabling negative behavior it seems to act in the opposite way. She knew as long as she allowed her daughter to stay, the young woman had a place to return after each mistreatment and argument until it blew over.

When this option was removed, her daughter was faced with a choice: either continue to live with the cycle of the man's abuse or begin to care for herself and admit she was being treated unacceptably. This was a choice only she could make. No matter how much my friend loved and cared for her, even as her mother, she was still powerless to change the behavior, perception, or self-esteem of her daughter.

At first the daughter was angry at having to move out of her mother's home. She felt abandoned and became distant and manipulative, blaming her mother when the relationship with her boyfriend spiraled out of control. But after living with her boyfriend, she had a change of heart.

My friend's daughter finally realized how she allowed herself to be mistreated by her boyfriend and his mother. Her mother's loving boundary helped open her heart to the reality of her situation. The young woman had to care enough for herself to finally say no to enabling further abuse.

It is a misconception to think we have the power to change other people. We may think an irresponsible person will mag-

CHAPTER 16

ically wake up if we are more understanding and patient; if we scream louder; if we are more logical or say it in a different way. This is not the case.

What changes us is choosing to live in line with our integrity. To love as Jesus did.

The truth is, our care and affection, no matter how deep, don't have the power to make other people change. Or get them to see reason. Or stop them from hurting us or themselves.

It was a hard-won lesson in personal integrity for my friend's daughter to accept the reality of her situation rather than the fantasy of what she thought the relationship could be. She chose to change the only person she had power over—herself. She left her boyfriend to raise her child with her sister's and mother's help. Through her mother's tough-love boundary, she learned what caring and affection really are as well as what they are not.

Her former boyfriend quickly moved on and got another girl pregnant. Just like my friend's daughter, until this man achieves a higher level of self-awareness and responsibility, he will not wake up to what it means to love. The reality may be that he never questions his actions. He may continue to be irresponsible. He may never learn that love is affection displayed as the positive behaviors of his integrity in action.

To live as ambassadors of Jesus-like love takes an enduring self-respect and care. We have to treat ourselves with the deep affection necessary to motivate ourselves to do the work required to constantly evaluate and control our behavior and to learn from and change the negative choices we make as soon as possible.

No one can do this deliberate and ongoing internal assessment for us. Each of us has to respect and value ourselves so we will want to wake up to the reality of how we are behaving. Choosing to be responsible for the consequences of our actions is one way we love and respect ourselves.

Love Has Excellent Vision

I was addicted to cigarettes for twenty-two years. One day I stopped smoking. No one helped me end this unhealthy habit. For over two decades, many people who cared deeply for me told me I had to quit. They constantly bombarded me with information about the harmful effects of cigarettes. But they could only encourage me to quit smoking.

I quit smoking because I chose to care for myself. I had to love myself awake to admit and take responsibility for the harmful effects of smoking. Stopping to question why I was harming myself was the only thing that provided the willpower I needed to stop picking up even one cigarette, ever again.

The same level of self-care was necessary for me to lose the fifty-three pounds I gained from attempting to stuff my emotions down. It also took deep self-love to stop gossiping, to stop being financially irresponsible, and to stop blaming people for the negatives in my life. Just as we must stop allowing others to mistreat us, we must also set boundaries against self-abuse.

Each day of life is a gift that provides experiences designed to teach us about ourselves and other people. When we reaffirm our responsible choices and learn from our mistakes, we are reborn, in a way. Each bad habit we transform allows us to deepen our connection to the integrity of our souls.

To create our best life, we strive to give the best of ourselves to life. We answer to ourselves for our behavior. And maybe like me, you also believe there is an all-powerful source to which we answer. I believe God is always with us and is aware of each beat of our heart. God is patient and allows us to learn. God forgives our mistakes when we accept responsibility for the impact of our hurtful behavior. God knows our requests for forgiveness are genuine when we care about the consequences of our actions.

How can we explain to God we did our best when we know we did not?

CHAPTER 16

When we behave with integrity, we bring the best of our character to all of our relationships, including the people we meet in coffee shops, in elevators, or on the street. We also bring the best of ourselves to situations in which no one else is involved.

I was walking my little dog, Ruby, when we came upon a shattered glass bottle. Sharp shards of clear glass were strewn several feet across the entire sidewalk. I carefully picked Ruby up and carried her around the glass. When we finished our walk and returned to the apartment, I got a broom, dustpan, and paper bag. I lined the bottom of the bag with a thick newspaper and in big red letters wrote "Careful, broken glass" on the outside of the bag. Then I headed to the next block with my cleanup tools in hand.

For about five minutes, I picked up the big pieces. I spent a few more minutes cleaning up the small shards that had fallen into the grass. I finished by sweeping the length of sidewalk and stairs leading up to the apartment where the bottle had broken.

As I returned home, I felt peaceful satisfaction. In taking time to clean up the glass, I realized the majority of my contentment with life comes from doing what I can to make a positive difference. It makes my heart sing to think I may have prevented even a single other person or an animal from being hurt.

When we understand love is the caring and affection of our integrity in action, our behavior can become the superhero power we use to create a world of respect, compassion, equality, and peace. We will no longer know bullying, abuse, war, or discrimination. We will stop persecuting one another because of skin color, sexuality, gender, politics, or religion. We can be ambassadors of Jesus-like love.

As ambassadors of Jesus's loving integrity, we can create a world where all life is respected and protected. A world where the freedom to speak and act is balanced by personal responsibility

Love Has Excellent Vision

for the consequences of our words and actions. A world where we openly and responsibly share our feelings. A world where we listen to one another to understand. A world where being a person of true character is the universal benchmark for success.

You and I most certainly can make the world a better place when we work to improve the only person whose behavior we can truly control or change: ours. When we strive to behave as an example of Jesus's love in action, our little part of the world will begin to change for the better. And one day in the not-too-distant future, all our little parts of the world will meet, and together we will have created a legacy we are proud to leave to our children and theirs.

17

Care about the Legacy We Leave

If we believe children are the future, then we must care about the legacy we are leaving. That requires us to understand the responsibility we have today to be a positive influence on our children's tomorrows.

I have two fathers. One is my biological father, Gene, who got my thirteen-year-old biological mother, Mary, pregnant. As you know, she gave me up for adoption.

My other father is my dad, Reagan, the man who raised me. As you also know, Jean (my mom) and Reagan could not have children, but they badly wanted a little one to share life with. So they adopted me.

I remember when Mom told me. I was about five years old, and we were sitting on the kitchen floor in our little house on Mistletoe Street in Victoria, Texas. She said I was deeply wanted and loved. So much so that she flew all the way to Plainview, Texas, to get me.

No matter what pain, rejection, and heartbreak I have shared about my early life, I don't remember a time when I did not feel like their child just because we lacked a biological connection. Love is not conditional. The love we have for one another is

Care about the Legacy We Leave

strong and forgiving. Over time, we healed our relationship. Today we love one another as Jesus wants us to.

During our decades together, I came to appreciate that you don't have to be special to father a child or bear a child. But to actually raise a child? That takes a daily commitment to do whatever is necessary to ensure the child feels love, acceptance, and self-worth as an individual; to teach the child to respect other people and all life; and to display for them the values of integrity and responsibility we want to pass on so they are equipped to create the best life possible.

Although my dad, Reagan, is far from perfect, just as I am, he is a man who chose to learn how to be a good father. My parents teamed up to show me how to live a life of responsibility, respect, and honesty. I am honored to have been adopted by them and am deeply grateful to have been parented by them.

Raising children is a huge job with a huge amount of personal responsibility. Children learn by watching their parents and other people with whom they associate. The greatest legacy we can give children is teaching them to be people of Jesus-like integrity and empathy.

I don't have children of my own, but I am blessed to have a godson, goddaughter, niece, and nephew. I also have many neighbors, friends, and family members with children of various ages. I think of all of those children maybe one day having children and grandchildren of their own, and on and on for generations. And this causes me to wonder what manner of life and world I am helping leave to them and the generations that come after.

Am I creating a masterpiece from my life I am proud to leave as an example to future generations?

Am I actively working to create or helping to destroy our children's future?

CHAPTER 17

No matter whether we are parents or not, as human beings we are all related, which means we are collectively responsible for the future of all children. I first embraced the reality of the connectedness of all life during my Inipi sweat lodge ceremony experience. I now know the importance of the generational respect Native peoples have. Each time we spoke or finished a prayer in the Inipi, our Lakota leader led us in saying "mitakuye oyasin," meaning "all my relations," or "all are related." We share a past, present, and future.

You will remember a DNA test confirmed my genetic relations all the way back to Cheddar man, who lived in the United Kingdom around 10,000 years ago. DNA testing has become an important tool for many of us who are interested in learning about our inherited makeup. Investigating our ancestry has also become big business as an increasing number of us want to know our connection to past relatives. In learning more about our origin stories, we can acknowledge our ancestors' sacrifices, honor the vast challenges they overcame, appreciate the accomplishments they contributed to make life easier and safer for us, and acknowledge their numerous mistakes.

The goal is to leave a kinder, equitable, and respectful world for our children. What would life be like if, as parents and nonparents alike, we started focusing on how the actions we take today are affecting all children, and theirs, and theirs?

I think this is an important question Jesus would want us to ask ourselves, because I believe he would feel out of place in our world. Not because of the ways we have advanced since the time in which he lived—I am certain he would embrace them as a way to share his heart with us in the style we are familiar with—but because he would not be able to wrap his heart around the fact

Care about the Legacy We Leave

that we, as a human family, have not significantly improved our collective spiritual maturity in two millennia.

Jesus would be disappointed, I am sure, that we, as a human family, don't appreciate the importance of respecting ourselves and all the world's women and men, children, and animals. He would not approve of continuous war and environmental destruction to gain control over the world's resources and establish dominance over others. He would not value those who allow greed to drive them. Moreover, he would be disgusted that women are still treated as second-class citizens; that we judge and dehumanize one another over skin color, sexual orientation, religion, or political party affiliation; and that we so easily surrender to the egocentric drive to dominate, divide, and destroy.

Jesus would remind us these behaviors don't align with the lessons he taught of humility and togetherness, of self-discipline over individualistic ego, and of having one's fair share without being selfish.

We must live to make Jesus and our children proud.

When you and I look honestly at the challenges we face, it is evident we, as Christians and professed lovers of Christ, have work to do. We need to accept that until we rise in energized harmony to productively address these challenges, Jesus will remain disappointed by the legacy we are leaving. But in addition to Jesus's discontent, unless we get our act together, we also will not be viewed kindly in the eyes and hearts of our children, who are pleading with us to lead the way to a better future.

I believe Jesus would tell us failing to care how our actions today are creating a bleak outlook for our children's tomorrow is failing to honor him and his sacrifice.

I believe Jesus would challenge us to consider why we are leav-

CHAPTER 17

ing the negative effects of social and political instability, environmental degradation, and gender inequality to our children, and theirs, to deal with.

I believe Jesus would direct us to wake up from our coma of self-induced apathy to responsibly acknowledge the impact our negative behavior is having on the generations to come—not just future humans, but all life that God created and wants us to nurture with care, respect, and responsibility.

And I don't think those beliefs are a stretch to anyone who has read the New Testament with an open heart.

The phrase *mitakuye oyasin* refers to more than just the people who came before. I agree with the Lakota and Native peoples who believe we are all related: our human family, the natural world, and those generations that come after us. Therefore, I believe Jesus would ask these questions of everyone who professes to love him:

> *Do we care about the ways our need for immediate gratification and our gluttony for the world's resources are affecting our children's future?*
> *Why don't we consider caring for the earth, for future generations, part of honoring Jesus's life and death?*
> *Judging from the chaos and environmental destruction in the world, doesn't it seem time for us to do things differently?*

Courage is what empowers a person to face struggles, pain, difficulty, and even the unknown. Some people would even argue it is what allows us to tackle those challenges without fear. Yes, when we are courageous, we bravely face danger and possible harm. However, I don't agree that acting courageously means we are not afraid, as I am confident Jesus was frightened to suffer and die.

Care about the Legacy We Leave

Gerome, my friend who went into the burning building to rescue the old man, told me he was afraid. My friend Peter was afraid to come to terms with the physical and mental abuse he endured from his alcoholic father. My friend Petric was terrified to testify against his uncle and the KKK White supremacists who bombed the Sixteenth Street Baptist Church. I was petrified to tell my parents I was gay. However, we did not let the fear of whatever uncertainty or intimidation we might encounter stop us from doing what we knew was right. Courage to do what is right comes from our souls.

Courage is a choice we make to willingly face physical pain, hardship, or the threat of death. It is a moral choice to take the right action in the face of popular opposition, discouragement, or personal loss.

What would the world look like if you and I truly honored Jesus and our children by courageously working to advance our soul's empathy and integrity?

I have not studied with a guru, master, or spiritual teacher. As you know, my early experience with organized religion took me off the path of following other people's beliefs and led me to forge my own trail. My heart teachers have been everyday people who gather the courage to overcome even the worst situations in order to make their lives better.

One of my most profound teachers was a young woman of about seventeen, whom I met when I was in my twenties. When she was raped by a man she considered a safe friend, her response was, "What do I have to learn from this horrible experience?"

My reaction at the time was, "What? Are you kidding me? How could anyone who is an innocent victim question herself after undergoing such a violent and traumatic experience?"

Obviously I was shocked and could not comprehend how she was not enraged or why she did not want revenge. At that time in

CHAPTER 17

life, as her friend, I could think of at least one hard and painful lesson the man needed to learn. After some time and conversation, however, I began to understand my friend was making the intentional choice to take an appalling situation—one she was powerless to have stopped or to now change—and turn it around to find what was within her power to do so she could move herself forward.

Witnessing the depth of her courage and mature level of self-reflection helped expand my soul. I began to appreciate that we make ourselves better, and therefore the lives of our children better, by growing our spiritual natures. We grow our souls by choosing to honestly look to ourselves and determine what we need to learn from the challenges we face and what we can do to move ourselves forward, which helps the world move forward no matter how awful it has been to us in the process.

We can transform ourselves, society, and our relationships for the better! I believe Jesus wants us to ask ourselves the questions and consider the observations I have raised in this book. Jesus would join us in bravely questioning the logic of falling in line with the beliefs and practices our ancestors have passed down without examining them thoughtfully first. We must love Jesus and honor his life and sacrifice by choosing to make better, wiser choices than the generations that came before us.

I did not choose the color of my skin or where I grew up, the religion I was exposed to, or the information I received in school. My parents, religion, and society did their best, as yours did, to mold me into who they wanted me to be. I learned early in life to question my thoughts, experiences, and other people's beliefs based on what felt right in my heart—the place where Jesus was supposed to dwell.

To honor Jesus, we have a responsibility to grow as the spiritual beings we are. The only obstacle standing between living

Care about the Legacy We Leave

from our spiritual nature or not is a choice—a choice to lead with logic and love and make right what we know Jesus would consider wrong about our attitudes, beliefs, and behavior.

What would our world look like if we chose to make this conversation the start of our to-do list in order to courageously rise up and create life differently from previous generations?

To love Jesus and one another, let's care about the legacy we are leaving for ourselves, other people, and the generations to come. Let's lead a labor of love and begin respectful but honest conversations among our family, friends, and church congregations about what we need to do to be right with Jesus. Let's seek out and join with like-hearted people, regardless of religious or political affiliation, who are actively working to create the positive change we all want to see. Let's join with people who are setting a responsible, kind, and respectful example of what it means to be a good global citizen.

Let's set aside our differences to focus on the common goal of doing everything within our power to create a better world than the one we are currently leaving to our descendants. It is not too late to make Jesus truly proud. He would remind us that by choosing to advance the souls we are, we will create a peaceful, respectful, and sustainable future for our children and theirs.

So how do we build this new world?

We act, today, as the superheroes God created us to be.

Acknowledgments

My heartfelt appreciation to Peggy Boatright; Kristen Cannata; Natalie Motise Davis, PhD; Brooke Fisher; Cindy Frost; Reverend Mike Harper; Rose Marie Higgins; Autumn Joy Jimerson; Joyce Leddel; Pat Lile; Jessica Gabrielle McKay; Barbara Simon; Vicki Walton; and Carolyn Wieczorek, for their time, loving support, and kindness in reviewing parts or all of the manuscript and providing valuable input.

I am deeply grateful to Caleb, Charles, Christopher, Crissy, David, Miguel, Sharmila, Shanti, Reverend Britt Skarda, and Reverend Timothy Moody for their contributions.

A big thank you to Tina Rubin and Tiffany Yecke Brooks, PhD, for their editing expertise and the vital part both played in helping transform the manuscript into this book.

I also want to thank Lisa Ann Cockrel, Trevor Thompson, and the publishing team at Wm. B. Eerdmans Publishing Company for having the confidence in the manuscript to take up this project.

To each of the people named above, and to others not acknowledged here, thank you. This book was several years in

ACKNOWLEDGMENTS

the making and involved the support of friends, family, and countless members of my heart family. This labor of love would not have found form without the contributions each made to this process.

Notes

Over my lifetime I have read hundreds of books and articles and listened to countless hours of lectures on a wide variety of topics. I am confident some of the knowledge I have gained from others has found its way onto the pages of this book, expressed in my unique voice. What follows highlights the specific books, articles, and websites I quoted from directly when writing *The Real Conversation Jesus Wants Us to Have*.

1. Brené Brown, *The Gifts of Imperfection* (Center City, MN: Hazelden Publishing, 2020), 10.
2. Quoted in David J. B. Krishef, "Ethics and Religion Talk: What Is a Legitimate Religious Practice?," *Rapidian* (blog), March 21, 2023, https://tinyurl.com/3nt7p9st.
3. Benjamin Cremer (@Brcremer), Twitter, June 6, 2023, https://tinyurl.com/2debrf7u.
4. John Shelby Spong, "Walking into the Mystery of God," Unitarian Universalist Association, November 12, 2015, https://tinyurl.com/2f8umyrs.
5. Matthew Vines, *God and the Gay Christian: The Biblical Case in Support of Same-Sex Relationships* (New York: Convergent, 2014).

6. Caleb Kaltenbach and Matthew Vines, "Debating Bible Verses on Homosexuality," *New York Times*, June 8, 2015, https://tinyurl.com/5cxvj9bc.

7. Steven Novella, "The Science of Biological Sex: What Does the Science Actually Say about Biological Sex?," *Science-Based Medicine* (blog), July 13, 2022, https://tinyurl.com/52sc4jw7.

8. Dick F. Swaab, "Sexual Orientation and Its Basis in Brain Structure and Function," *Proceedings of the National Academy of Sciences of the United States of America*, July 29, 2008, https://tinyurl.com/39xnm9zb.

9. Elliot Kukla, "Ancient Judaism Recognized a Range of Genders. It's Time We Did Too," *New York Times*, March 18, 2023.

10. Quoted in David Nichols, "Pastoral Ponderings . . . ," https://tinyurl.com/yeyret3n, accessed February 2024.

11. "The Bible," History.com editors, updated April 23, 2019, https://tinyurl.com/yj98pkf3.

12. Emily Swan and Ken Wilson, *Solus Jesus: A Theology of Resistance* (Canton, MI: Read the Spirit, 2018), 38–39, 44.

13. Quoted in James F. McGrath, "Not Liberal, Just Literate," *Patheos*, November 26, 2016, https://tinyurl.com/z6uw3rrp.

14. Jennifer Butler, "The Heresy of Christian Nationalism," Red Letter Christians, January 19, 2022, https://tinyurl.com/27dtmzyf.

15. Swan and Wilson, *Solus Jesus*, 187.

16. Regina Cates, *Lead with Your Heart: Creating a Life of Love, Compassion and Purpose* (San Antonio, TX: Hierophant, 2014).

17. Dalai Lama, Facebook, September 7, 2010, https://tinyurl.com/yckxdpm2.

18. Swan and Wilson, *Solus Jesus*, 273–74.

19. C. S. Lewis, "The Problem of Evil and the Necessity of Choice," C. S. Lewis Institute, August 2007, https://tinyurl.com/445jdvte.

20. Kyshaun Drakes, "MCU: The Strongest and Weakest Members of the Avengers," Screen Rant, May 4, 2022, https://tinyurl.com/2jfpneba.

21. John Zerzan, "Patriarchy, Civilization, and the Origins of Gender," The Anarchist Library, April 13, 2010, https://tinyurl.com/5abyytj2.

22. Leonard Shlain, *Sex, Time, and Power: How Women's Sexuality Shaped Human Evolution* (London: Penguin, 2003), 337–39.

23. Michael Hall, "Politicians in Black Robes," *Texas Monthly*, September 2022, 121–23, 192–97.

24. Brian Duignan, "Federalist Society," *Britannica*, March 20, 2021, https://tinyurl.com/3zb68d42.

25. Elie Mystal, "The U.S. Constitution Was Meant to Be a Work in Progress," interview by Sonali Kolhatkar, *Yes!*, March 2022, https://tinyurl.com/5n89hkmz.

26. Mystal, "U.S. Constitution."

27. Quoted in Destinee Adams, "I Hated History—until I Learned about Shirley Chisholm," National Public Radio, March 22, 2024, https://tinyurl.com/4ykep7a5.

28. Mary Daly, *Beyond God the Father: Toward a Philosophy of Women's Liberation* (Boston: Beacon, 1973).

29. Swan and Wilson, *Solus Jesus*, 38–39.

30. "The 2003 Pulitzer Prize Winner in Public Service," The Pulitzer Prizes, https://tinyurl.com/56thhzzk.

31. Kate Shellnut, "Southern Baptists Refused to Act on Abuse, Despite Secret List of Pastors," *Christianity Today*, May 22, 2022, https://tinyurl.com/3eztjnwa.

32. Russell Moore, "This Is the Southern Baptist Apocalypse," *Christianity Today*, May 22, 2022, https://tinyurl.com/yhsk3brc.

33. Quoted in Lindsey Lanquist, "Watch This Nun Explain Ex-

actly What It Means to Be Pro-Life," Self.com, July 2017, https://tinyurl.com/4nny62y4.

34. Lisa Green, "New Survey: Women Go Silently from Church to Abortion Clinic," CareNet.org, November 23, 2015, https://tinyurl.com/ba9hhruh.

35. Sandee LaMotte, "Myths about Abortion and Women's Mental Health Are Widespread, Experts Say," CNN, July 3, 2022, https://tinyurl.com/3w9jvmxz.

36. LaMotte, "Myths about Abortion."

37. Shlain, *Sex, Time and Power*, 337–39.

38. Quoted in Charles Pierce, "Politics Don't Corrupt People. People Corrupt Politics," *Esquire*, December 18, 2019, https://tinyurl.com/5dzb28wy.

39. Heather Cox-Richardson, *Letters to an American*, Substack, February 15, 2023.

40. Quoted in Tara Isabella Burton, "The Biblical Story the Christian Right Uses to Defend Trump," *Vox*, March 5, 2018, https://tinyurl.com/bdaak9t4.

41. Swan and Wilson, *Solus Jesus*, 202.

42. David Fastenow, "Our Common Beliefs," letter to the editor, in *Arkansas-Democrat Gazette*, November 5, 2017.

43. Max Boot, "The Supreme Court Rulings Represent the Tyranny of the Minority," *Washington Post*, June 25, 2022, https://tinyurl.com/3vc7swnu.

44. Mickey Edwards, "How to Turn Republicans and Democrats into Americans," *Atlantic*, July/August 2011, https://tinyurl.com/5n7dw2zc.

45. Brett Hennig, *The End of Politicians: Time for a Real Democracy* (London: Unbound, 2017).

46. Robert Reich, "The Stadium Scam," Substack, February 11, 2023.

Notes to Pages 132–152

47. Rebekah Sager, "Guess Who's behind the 'He Gets Us' Commercials That Ran During the Superbowl?," *Daily Kos*, February 13, 2023, https://tinyurl.com/4myjzecb.

48. Sarah Pruitt, "The Ongoing Mystery of Jesus's Face," History.com, updated March 18, 2024, https://tinyurl.com/bvnpem6c.

49. Debby Irving, *Waking Up White and Finding Myself in the Story of Race* (Plano, TX: Elephant Room, 2014), 153.

50. Debby Irving, "Are Prejudice, Bigotry, and Racism the Same Thing?," DebbyIrving.com, https://tinyurl.com/5xms8kyu, accessed May 2020.

51. Quoted in Jena McGregor, "The Most Memorable Passage in George W. Bush's Speech Rebuking Trumpism," *Washington Post*, October 20, 2017, https://tinyurl.com/3tj5duby.

52. Theodore R. Johnson, "We Used to Count Black Americans as 3/5 of a Person," *Washington Post*, August 21, 2015, https://tinyurl.com/3v722sm2.

53. Ileana Najarro, "Florida's New African American History Standards: What's behind the Backlash," *Education Week*, July 25, 2023, https://tinyurl.com/35h98u25.

54. Mashama Bailey and John O. Morisano, *Black, White, and the Grey: The Story of an Unexpected Friendship and a Beloved Restaurant* (New York: Lorena Jones, 2021), 117.

55. Joy DeGruy, *Post Traumatic Slave Syndrome: America's Legacy of Enduring Injury and Healing* (Portland, OR: Joy DeGruy Publications, 2017), 173.

56. Irving, *Waking Up White*, 35.

57. Michelle Alexander, *The New Jim Crow: Mass Incarceration in the Age of Colorblindness* (New York: New Press, 2011), 1–2.

58. Elie Mystal, *Allow Me to Retort: A Black Guy's Guide to the Constitution* (New York: New Press, 2022); Nikole Hannah-Jones, Caitlin

Roper, Ilena Silverman, and Jake Silverstein, eds., *The 1619 Project: A New Origin Story* (New York: One World, 2021).

59. James King, *The Biology of Race* (Oakland: University of California Press, 1981), 118.

60. DeGruy, *Post Traumatic Slave Syndrome*, 118.

61. Michaela Brenner and Vincent Hearing, "The Protective Role of Melanin against UV Damage in Human Skin," US National Library of Medicine, National Institutes of Health, May 2009, https://tinyurl.com/pzxsy6mf.

62. Quoted in "Atomic Education Urged by Einstein; Scientist in Plea for $200,000 to Promote New Type of Essential Thinking," *New York Times*, May 25, 1946, 11, https://tinyurl.com/3uh3e684.

63. Robert Reich, "Resilience," October 29, 2021, Substack.